TANTRA

The Path to

Blissful

Sex

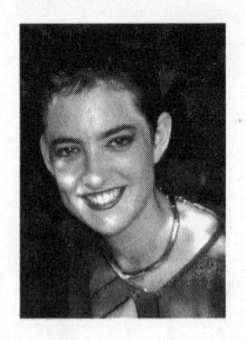

ABOUT THE AUTHOR

Leora Lightwoman has been teaching Tantra since 1995. Before this, Leora obtained her MA (Hons) degree in psychology from Oxford University, and trained and worked as a yoga teacher and massage therapist. She began practising Tantra in Australia with Tantric/Shamanic teachers at the Centre for Human Transformation. Thereafter, Leora received further tuition in Tantra and Native American sexuality teachings from various teachers around the world, and proceeded to complete the SkyDancing USA Tantra Teachers' Training with Margot Anand. Leora is also qualified in voice dialogue, a meditative and therapeutic technique for unifying the different aspects of ourselves, and as a holistic breathwork therapist. She has trained in couples' counselling, and is currently completing her training as a body psychotherapist.

Having developed her own approach to Tantra, Leora set up her Tantra school, Diamond Light Tantra, in 2000. She runs workshops and courses throughout the UK and abroad, and offers private Tantra sessions for women and couples in London. Leora's particular gifts include her capacity to share her depth of understanding of Tantra and human psychology in a safe, accessible, meaningful and enjoyable way. Her advanced workshops are co-facilitated by her husband, Dr Roger Lichy.

Visit the Piatkus website!

Piatkus publishes a wide range of bestselling fiction and non-fiction, including books on health, mind, body and spirit, sex, self-help, cookery, biography and the paranormal.

If you want to:
- read descriptions of our popular titles
- buy our books over the internet
- take advantage of our special offers
- enter our monthly competition
- learn more about your favourite Piatkus authors

VISIT OUR WEBSITE AT: www.piatkus.co.uk

Copyright © 2004 by Leora Lightwoman

First published in Great Britain in 2004 by
Piatkus Books Ltd
5 Windmill Street, London W1T 2JA
email: info@piatkus.co.uk

The moral right of the author has been asserted

A catalogue record for this book is available from the British Library

ISBN 0 7499 2473 X

Edited by Krystyna Mayer
Text design by Two Associates
Illustrations by Sharon Waxkirsh

This book has been printed on paper manufactured
with respect for the environment using wood from
managed sustainable resources

Typeset by Action Publishing Technology Ltd, Gloucester
Printed and bound in Great Britain by MPG Books, Bodmin, Cornwall

TANTRA

The Path to
Blissful
Sex

LEORA LIGHTWOMAN

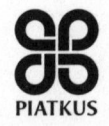

PIATKUS

CONTENTS

Acknowledgements vii
Introduction ix
List of techniques xvii

1. The Tantric journey 1
2. First steps 10
3. Delicious beginnings for couples 28
4. Tantra alone and as a single person 47
5. Intimate relationship as a spiritual path 60
6. Tantric principles in lovemaking and life 78
7. The chakra system 100
8. Meeting your chakras 115
9. Male and female energy flow 128
10. Opening to love 149
11. Opening to pleasure 160
12. Shakti mysteries 177
13. Shiva wisdom 193
14. Our sacred sexual organs 208
15. Sacred union: integrating sex, love, relationship and spirit . . . 229

Resources 250
Index 252

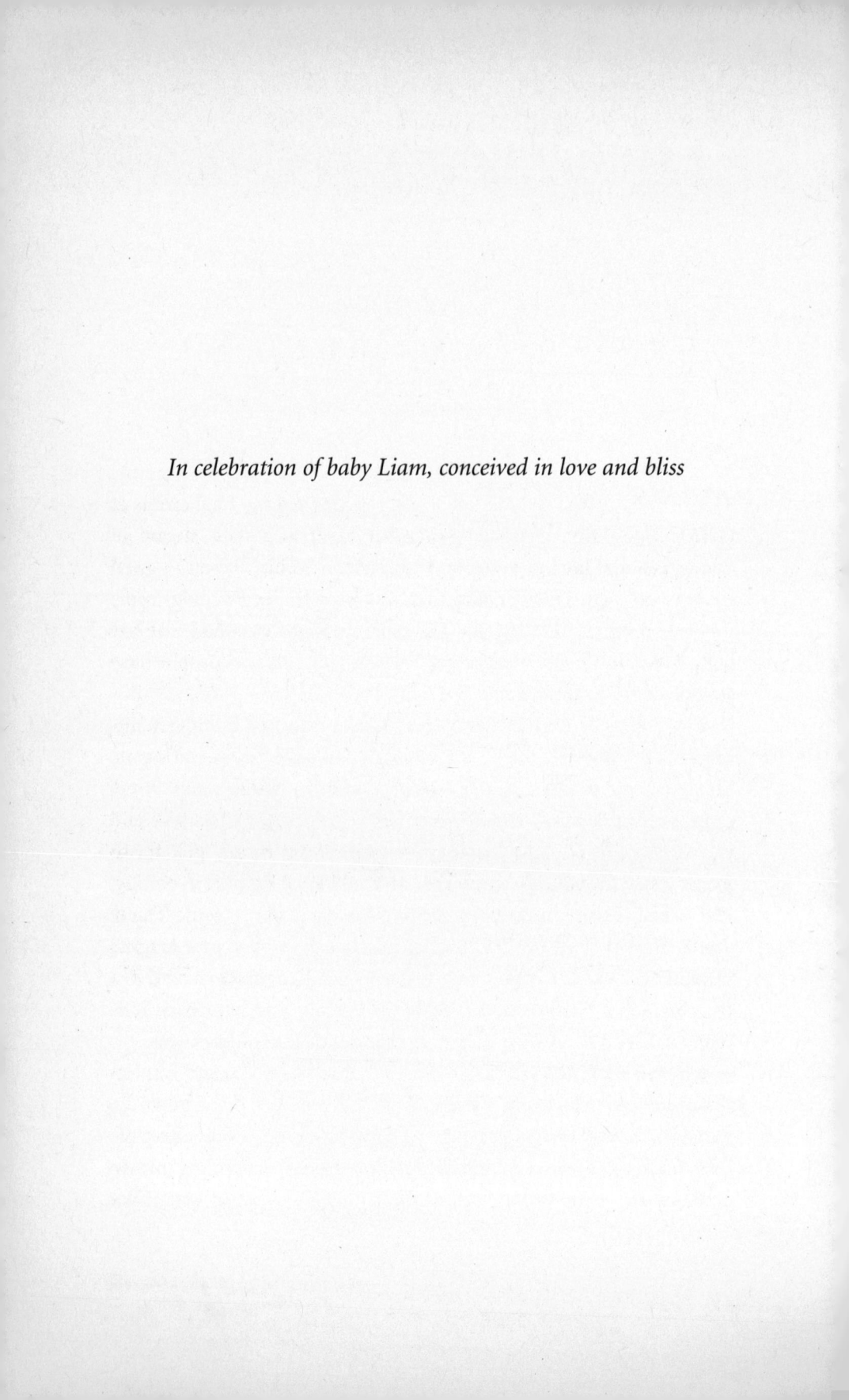

In celebration of baby Liam, conceived in love and bliss

ACKNOWLEDGEMENTS

Twelve years before writing this book, I completed my final exams at Oxford University, absolutely burnt out after an endless stream of essay crises and life in the fast lane of academic achievement. I vowed never to go back. Transforming that past experience of writing-from-the-head into manifesting my vision of writing-from-the-heart has been a beautiful and challenging odyssey, and many people have supported me in this journey.

I would like to thank Steve Nobel for propelling me into the manifestation of this book, and wise woman Rosy Daniel for mentoring me through some of the ups and downs of writing. All blessings to my special friend Natalie Dorchester for being genuinely enthusiastic and encouraging, at all times, from your heart. I am hugely grateful to Annie Evans for your no-nonsense, slash and burn support in editing, and to Sally Fraser for keeping me to the essence of my work. Thank you to Sharon Waxkirsh for crossing continents to offer your magical illustrations, and for staying with it even when it looked like we'd lost the plot. Anna Crago and Gill Bailey at Piatkus, you have been infinitely patient and trusting on many, many occasions – thank you.

I have been gifted with many great teachers, mentors, and inspirational guides in the manifestation of the Tantric work that I teach. To name but a few, Margot Anand and John Hawken for launching me into teaching, Helena Lovendal for continually reminding me to embrace my own power and authority, and, together with Nick

Duffell, for your gender psychology teachings. Thank you to Sarita and Geho for the breast and vajra meditations. I am immensely grateful to all my Tantra workshop participants, individual clients, colleagues and friends for your ongoing teachings. Special thanks to those of you who have offered quotes and personal stories, many of which, through lack of space, have not been included in the final version, but remain in my heart. You have generously shared your riches with others, and without you I could not have written this book.

My retreat into intimate relationship with my computer has clearly affected, and relied upon the support of those in my daily life. Without the commitment, vision, love, humour, inspired work, and many late nights of Aida Capelli, my manager, and the ongoing support of Teertha Ordish, my administrator, the running of Diamond Light Tantra in my absence would not have happened. Jon Lightman, my brother and 'legal angel', I could not have done without when confronted with daunting paperwork. Robin Baldock has been a wonderfully dedicated friend and colleague in all sorts of ways, helping workshops to go ahead amidst my crazy juggling of priorities. My mother, Elaine Lightman, arranged and financed several 'writing retreats' in luxurious locations, allowing me to be creative in true Tantric style. Love, gratitude and blessings to you all. Thank you too to friends Libby Forsyth and Alexia Severis for sharing your homes and your inner warmth.

My beloved husband, and fellow explorer of the mysteries of Tantra, Roger Lichy, has lived with a sleep-deprived and preoccupied author for a whole year. Thank you for dragging me away from my desk to eat and relate, and to your dedicated sperm for finding the perfect moment, amidst manuscripts, to conceive our wondrous baby.

INTRODUCTION

This book is both for couples and individuals, for people embarking on the journey of Tantra and for those who have already set sail. It is for lovers and would-be lovers of life of all ages who have a genuine desire to look deeply into themselves. It is for those who have the willingness to let go of trodden paths in order to make way for perceiving new worlds that were always there, hiding beneath the surface.

Tantra is primarily about uniting love and sexuality with awareness. Tantra is about loving ourselves. It is also a celebration of the flow of loving sexuality between two people. Through allowing this sexual love to deepen and expand, an opening may arise to experience ecstasy.

Tantra is recognising that deepest, truest place in all whom we meet. It is a moment when we are totally absorbed in awe with the beauty of nature, music or art. Tantra is about truly loving and embracing all of life, and through this love remembering our essence, the divine.

ROOTS AND MEANING OF TANTRA

The word 'Tantra' comes from Sanskrit roots and means 'weaving' and 'expansion'. We can understand this to mean that when we fully accept (weave together) all aspects of life, our horizons expand so that we perceive and experience life more fully and joyfully.

Tantra is thought to have originated in India around 3,500 years ago, when the Aryans invaded northern India. The indigenous Dravidian culture, which had worshipped the earth as a feminine expression of creative energy, was replaced by a masculine, sun-worshipping religion of its conquerors. Tantra is thought to have developed as a synthesis of these two opposing influences. The exact time when Tantra began is hard to trace; rather than emerging as a school, it originated among individual spiritual practitioners and was passed down orally from a lineage of masters (many of whom were women) to their disciples. Tantra became manifest, in the form of Tantric scriptures, the Tantras, only in the eighth century AD. Many of these writings took the form of discourses between divine lovers. A central icon of Tantra was the sexual and spiritual union of the masculine and feminine principles or archetypal deities, Shiva (male deity, who also represents pure consciousness) and Shakti (female deity, who also represents pure energy).

Whereas the prevailing Hindu religion was dominated by very strict rules and the caste system, Tantra was available to everyone, both men and women, from the lowest castes to royalty. Tantric rituals emerged that directly broke all of the major taboos in Hinduism, in order to liberate the energy locked away in a rigid mindset. By breaking out of perceived limitations to behaviour, the mind was given a wider vantage point for viewing reality. It is a myth, however, to associate Tantra only with exotic sexual practices, as this is only one expression of a wide-ranging panoply of meditations, guided by a realistic and beautiful attitude to life and spiritual practice.

Tantric strands were later assimilated into Hinduism and Buddhism, and took on qualities of these religions. Tantra itself, however, is not a religion, but a direct expression of universal truths that require no particular belief system or cultural trappings.

Tantra does not require complicated postures, a vegetarian diet or even an affinity with Eastern religious thought. Tantra is not even a philosophy, as it neither requires any previous beliefs, nor advocates any. It simply offers a series of tools, tried and tested over the ages, to help us experience truth and freedom directly. I like to think of it as a process of remembering who we really are.

Tantra is essentially about unity. Instead of focusing on an afterlife of Heaven or Hell, it focuses on direct realisation of the divine, our pure and illuminated essential true nature, here and now. Tantra does not distinguish between the sacred and the profane. In direct contrast to religious practices that focus on asceticism, Tantra embraces the passions and the senses as tools that can be harnessed for transformation. It focuses on energy rather than structure. The emphasis is inwards, in extracting the medicine from the plants of life, for spiritual realisation.

WHAT IS TANTRA?

I shall first briefly elucidate what Tantra is not, or not just. It is not a variety of kinky sex; it does not involve candlelit orgies or wife-swapping parties. Tantra is not just a flavour of sex; blissful sex is an aspect of Tantra. Tantric techniques, in and of themselves, will not transform you into a super-lover, unless you are willing to change from the inside out. Tantra is not about better sexual performance; instead it is about profoundly more fulfilling and joyful sex, and a deeper and more enriching experience of life as a whole.

Tantra can mean many different things to different people, and its significance to one individual may evolve and change over time. Colin, a university lecturer, tells me, 'Tantra for me is about making love in a whole new way, enjoying sensuality, relaxing and having fun. It's about rediscovering my innocence.' 'Tantra is about intimacy and honest communication,' says his girlfriend.

The techniques in Tantra are many and varied. They may consist of anything from passionate lovemaking with your partner to silent meditation alone. Each is an opportunity for getting to know yourself more deeply, and to recognise your deeper, ecstatic potential.

Tantra helps us to reconnect with ourselves, and with our essential goodness. It can help us to find greater meaning in our lives. When our own inner light shines brightly, other people are free to believe, feel and behave as they choose, and we remain rooted like a tree, with our topmost leaves swaying blissfully in the breeze.

Tantra is the art and science of energy. It shows us how to move energy inside and beyond the physical body, harnessing the enormous force of sexual desire. In this way, sex becomes far more than just a genital event. It can be a form of exquisite and intimate communication at many levels, simultaneously a deeply relaxing and a scintillatingly sensual experience. Sexual loving may be a source of replenishment and reconnection with ourselves, the Universe, our essence.

Tantra is also about awareness. It is about fully inhabiting your body when you make love, and the rest of the time too! *'While I was receiving pleasure from my partner,'* says Belinda, *'I kept thinking of all the things I should be doing, like seeing to the kids and doing the laundry.'* This kind of experience is very common. Many of us spend our lives with our minds and bodies inhabiting rather different worlds. In contrast, to be fully present in each moment is Tantra.

> *After the Tantric meditation, neither my partner nor I wanted to speak. There was a delicious quality of silence and intimacy between us. We had both been so absolutely engaged with each other throughout, that although I could hardly remember what had actually happened, it didn't really matter. All I needed to know was that it was beautiful, magical and special.*
>
> GEORGE, 38, LIBRARIAN

Tantra invites us into the magical world of the present via the physical body, called in Tantra the 'Temple of the Spirit'. Whereas our minds are constantly reflecting on the past and planning for the future, our body is here and now. Through entering deeply into the experience of embodiment, of physicality, we can transcend physical limitations and experience energy, bliss, ecstasy, truth.

Our bodies don't lie. Most cases of premature ejaculation, for example, are not, in my experience, the fault of any organic 'problem'. Instead, they are the body's honest and appropriate response to a range of emotional and relational issues, both from the man's personal history and in his current circumstances.

Tantra is a way out of the maze of the mind, leading us back to the simple truth of the body.

TANTRA AS A PATH OF HEALING

Many people assume that sexual interest and fulfilment decrease with the age of a relationship. *'We've come to see if Tantra can help us revamp our sex life. We've been together a long time though – over six years – so I guess that's normal.'* This statement, with a few variations, could easily have been uttered by nearly a quarter of the couples who come to see me. With some sexual and relationship healing, this need not be the case.

> *After thirty-six years together, my husband is still my best friend, and now, with Tantra, he has become an exquisite lover too.*
>
> ANGELA, 54, TEACHER

Sexual healing is desperately needed. Childhood sexual abuse is a horrible extreme in a whole spectrum of loss of innocence pervading the modern world. Most of us, whether we had a 'normal' childhood or not, could have benefited enormously from having our sexuality welcomed, appropriately and joyfully, by our parents.

As a toddler, what happened when you started to investigate your genitals? Was it a pleasurable, joyful discovery? Or were you told 'Don't do THAT!'? As a pubescent girl, when you had your first period, did you tell your mother? Did she congratulate you and welcome you into the mysteries of womanhood? As an adolescent boy, could you talk to your father, openly and honestly, about how to make love with a woman? Were your parents truly comfortable with their own sexuality, and able to convey to you the naturalness and beauty of corporal existence by being living examples of that truth? If you were not one of the lucky few, how do you imagine that your history continues to influence you now?

It is never too late to start again. Once we can acknowledge and grieve for what we once missed, our innate innocence is always here, not far beneath the surface, waiting to emerge. Sexual healing can range from changing our attitudes towards ourselves and our bodies, to choosing appropriate boundaries or receiving nurturing physical contact.

Our hearts and our genitals are two facets of the same jewel. Hurt one, and you cloud the brilliance of the other. Heal one, and you enhance the potential of the other. Feelings are what make us alive. To quote Chuck Spezzano, a visionary modern spiritual teacher, if you won a million pounds and didn't feel anything, all that money wouldn't mean anything to you. Tantra is simultaneously about opening our hearts, embracing our feelings and becoming more sensual.

TANTRIC TERMINOLOGY

The words that we choose to represent ourselves, our bodies and our sexuality will both reflect and reinforce how we see ourselves. For this reason, in Tantra we have the opportunity to use words that reflect our highest potential, words that inspire and connote beauty and sacredness. I shall be including these words throughout the book. Most importantly:

1. For 'vagina', I use the word 'yoni', meaning 'sacred place'.
2. For 'penis', I use the word 'vajra', meaning 'diamond thunderbolt' or 'unshakeable clarity'. Another word that is in fact more commonly used in Tantric texts is 'lingam', representing the universal male principle.
3. At times, for man or men, I use the word 'Shiva'. Shiva is the central male figure in Tantra, representing the enlightened, full potential of a male.

4. At times, for woman or women, I use the word 'Shakti'. Shakti, in Tantric texts, is the enlightened consort of Shiva, the female aspect of the Divine.

In your own private life, you may choose whatever words work for you, or make up your own. Simply be aware of whether your language supports or hinders you in celebrating the wonder, magic and beauty, the shining potential in you, your body and your sexuality.

HOW TO USE THIS BOOK

This book takes you through a process, a journey, with Tantra, in a progression that has been tried, tested and endorsed by many people. I suggest therefore that you engage in the exercises, meditations and practices basically in order. Do at least one practice from each chapter before progressing to the next. There's always a temptation, in a book like this one, to skip straight to the juicy bits nearer the end. Whereas you may choose to do this, I'd recommend acquiring a basis and context for the deeper work first.

Many of the themes and meditations are illustrated by personal accounts. I offer these accounts as a means to bring alive some of the wide variety of experiences that Tantra can give rise to. They are not examples of the 'right' way to respond, because in fact there is no right response to any exercise, except what you yourself discover about you. My hope is also that these stories impart a flavour of different individuals' journeys with Tantra, and that the same exercise or meditation practised at different junctures may yield entirely different results.

Several of the exercises are specifically for love partners. Most of these are just as applicable to same-sex couples as to heterosexual lovers. Some aspects of Tantric relating are, however, gender-specific, like the male/female breath. In these instances same-sex couples will need to include what is helpful and let go of what is irrelevant for them.

There are plenty of practices, in particular many of the foundation exercises, that can be done alone, and these are annotated (see the list on page xix). I would also recommend, at some stage, participating in a workshop programme (details are in the resources section, page 250) or both, in addition.

Please bear in mind that Tantra is a life path, a journey to be relished, rather than a goal to be achieved. You don't get any extra points for being first to arrive at the finishing line, so you might as well relax and enjoy the ride. I recommend interspersing time periods, say of a month or two, when you devote time to Tantric practice, with similar spans of time when you're not so disciplined, and simply allow what you have experienced to integrate in its own way into your life.

> *We were on holiday, making love. I looked into Larry's eyes and said, 'I've never experienced you like this before.' He smiled back at me and said, 'And I've never seen you in this way either.' It was both a simple and an immensely magical moment. After three years of practising Tantra, I felt that we had just begun.*
>
> SANDRA AND LARRY, 44 AND 57,
> SOCIAL WORKER AND COMPANY DIRECTOR

LIST OF TECHNIQUES

Some of the exercises, rituals, techniques and meditations listed below can be done as a single person, and some are to be done with a partner. Those suitable for one person are annotated with an S.

Exercise	Page
Namaste S	25
Melting hug	30
Back-to-back dance	33
Back-to-back dance: meeting your partner	34
Fingertip heart dance	36
Sensory awakening ritual	41
Inner love meditation S	49
Kundalini shaking S	53
Receptive gaze S	63
Eye gazing	65
Deep listening	67
Awareness in life S	80
Full body breathing S	87
Pelvic rocking meditation S	93
Sound in life: expressive sound meditation S	95
Meeting your love muscle S	116
Chakra breathing meditation S	118
Chakra talk S	125

The male breath S	135
The female breath S	137
The male–female breath	143
The body love ritual alone S	151
Body love ritual with friends	153
The 'yes, no, maybe and please' exercise	163
The yin–yang meditation	168
Uncovering pleasure-limiting belief systems	171
Tantric touch	174
The Shah! exercise S	179
Advanced Shah! exercise	181
Breast massage S	185
Breast meditation S	187
Admiring yoni S	188
Yoni gazing	190
Coming out of the cave: men's massage	200
Vajra meditation S	202
Vajra root meditation S	205
Self-love and self-pleasuring S	211
The hands are extensions of the heart massage	215
Shakti's delight	219
Shiva's delight	224
The heart wave, part 1: meeting	235
The heart wave, part 2: exchange	239
The wave of bliss, part 1: meditation	242
The wave of bliss, part 2: expansion	245

CHAPTER ONE

THE TANTRIC JOURNEY

I arrived at my first Tantric workshop, rather shyly and nervously, with a longing to establish a long-term, meaningful, integrated sexual, loving and spiritual relationship with a man. Previously I'd had most of these components separately in my life, but I'd never experienced all of them together in the same package.

I was at that time engaged in a five-year relationship with a Japanese Buddhist style of yoga, which I had also been teaching for the last two years. My yogic practice gave me a sense of meaning and a spiritual perspective on life. However, the range of my yoga teachings stopped short of mentioning the role of sexual relationships on the spiritual path. Noticeable by its absence, I could only assume that sex was either too banal or too profound a topic to be relevant to amateur yoginis like myself.

My boyfriend at the time was highly charged sexually, and we had a lot of fun together. Although I rarely had orgasms, and never during sexual intercourse, I had come to accept this as 'normal' for me, and did not really see it as a problem. So, having a boyfriend who loved my body and was keen on trying new things was very exciting and freeing for me. However, despite knowing that my boyfriend and I clearly loved each other, I found that I experienced our love most keenly during the overtures to sex, as well as when we were dancing, talking and eating together, rather than when we were actually making love. During lovemaking, my mind was very busy with a variety of highly engaging pursuits, such as finding the most pleasurable sensations, movements and positions, and hoping that my boyfriend would stay at it and in them for long enough to eventually take me over the edge into orgasm.

While all this was going on, my heart hardly ever had enough space or attention for its gentle voice to be heard. I was not aware that I longed for a greater sense of connectedness, of really feeling my boyfriend's love through sex, or that I was tired of having to work so hard at it all. So, although according to my modest expectations at the time I was sexually satisfied, at the end of our frenzies of passion I was often left feeling empty and alone, wondering what was wrong with me. My boyfriend was happy with how things were, and he saw no need to look further or more deeply than beneath the bedclothes, and so it was alone that I ventured into the world of Tantra.

Although I'd been taught that spiritual evolution was a long, slow and sometimes painful process, by the end of that first two-hour-long Tantra workshop, lights were flashing in more places than simply inside my underwear. Fully clothed and in a room full of strangers, I had glimpsed a simple, sensual, loving and expansive closeness with others and towards myself that was both personal and impersonal, completely new and yet strangely familiar.

What had I actually done to arrive in this exalted place? What stand out in my memory are moments when time stood still; a simple 'melting hug', an embrace that was probably as long as I'd ever held a lover in stillness. I remember dancing while focusing my awareness in my pelvis, simply for my own pleasure. I recall looking around with the eyes of a child who had just discovered a new and wonderful toy, and meeting the eyes of other innocent, shy and playful children all experimenting with the same joyful and exhilarating game. I remember gazing into another person's eyes and finding a place beyond words, sensing that we'd somehow been here together before.

PRACTISING TANTRA

In the 1990s, Tantra was only just starting to 'come out' in the West, and particularly in the UK, and dinner party conversations, not to mention family gatherings, were a little challenging for me. The word 'Tantra' was met with blank stares and polite little smiles, and occasionally someone would have the courage to ask 'What's that?' Nowadays, declaring my profession to those outside of the Tantra world is far more risky. 'Ohhh!' is a common response, 'You mean Tantric SEX!' Eyeballs roll and with mind whirring at top speed, images of orgies and outlandish sexual positions, marathon lovefests and masterful semen retention flood in. Despite their delight at such a riveting topic of conversation, complete with the chance to vicariously sample a flavour of forbidden fruits, they themselves wouldn't be seen dead pursuing such pleasures publicly.

It is partly in response to the private needs of individuals and couples to experience greater intimate and sexual fulfilment, together with a sense of spiritual connectedness, that I have written this book. My vision is that exploring Tantra at home with the support of a realistic and practical guidebook will be an immensely enjoyable and enriching experience for you.

I would be surprised, however, if at some point down the line, a little 'Tantric top-up' wouldn't go amiss. It would be misleading for me to suggest that every second of Tantric practice will inevitably be an experience of Divine bliss. If you imagined that to be the case, the moment an earthly feeling of discontent were to arise, you'd either conclude that Tantra 'didn't work', or that you were somehow, unlike the more enlightened beings among us, incapable of successfully entering the realms of ecstasy. I myself have felt like a failure many times, only to hear myself say, while teaching Tantra to others, 'You can't get it wrong!' At any given moment you will either be experiencing new levels of pleasure, love and bliss, or you will be getting to know more clearly what stops you from being there. In fact, it is common that when we feel most stuck and dissatisfied in our practice of Tantra, this is often the heralding of an important breakthrough into a new and greater level of freedom, aliveness and joy.

For this reason I wish to widen the context of the Tantric journey beyond the four walls of your bedroom, and to suggest that you at least consider, at some point, joining a workshop, forming a support group or seeking out some personal support or tuition as an individual or couple.

Writer and workshop leader Sobonfu Some, a woman who grew up in the West African Dagara tribe, teaches that within her culture it was understood that it would take the whole village to support each marital relationship. Practical skills, ceremonies and initiations, both for the couple and within the community, supported this vision. I am deeply touched and inspired by the degree of reverence that the ongoing journey of coupledom holds in the Dagara tribe. I believe that this is something that our throw-away culture of immediate gratification could benefit from considering. A symptom of our isolationist society is that we imagine we should always be able to do everything on our own. Why not give yourself a break and open to the beauty of recognising a wider community of like-minded people and supportive guides?

It is not necessary to have a partner to do Tantra. We were all born from the sexual union of our parents and this means that we are inherently sexual beings, whether or not we're having regular sex. What we do with our sexuality is only part of the issue; Tantra also encourages us to look at how we feel and how we choose to live with being intrinsically sexual.

How we are with our sexuality inevitably has consequences. If we expend a lot of energy keeping 'sex' tightly guarded in a cage, we are fighting ourselves. We will live in fear of it breaking out, and when it does, it is likely to be wild and untamed. We can never kill our basic nature. Alternatively, we can enjoy and acknowledge our sexuality, and choose an appropriate way to share it with the world. One creative and possibly Tantric expression of celibate sexuality is quoted in Nancy Friday's book *Women on Top*, when a nun, in response to the question of how she engages with her sexuality, replies: 'I pray naked.' When we feel at peace and in love within ourselves, a partner is an optional extra, or simply the icing on the cake.

A teacher of sexuality I knew once said, 'Sex for me is wonderful. It's the relationship bit that I find difficult!' This 'third being', the relationship, has a life of its own. In general, if we stick at a relationship for long enough, it will start with a 'honeymoon' phase (which feels wonderful), and evolve into a 'power struggle' or conflict stage (which doesn't feel so nice), before it has the possibility of transforming into a phase of transformation, where the two partners have a chance to meet on a new, deeper level. This cycle may repeat itself several times over the lifespan of an ongoing relationship. Tantra offers tools to support couples at all stages of this process.

Tantra, whether alone or with a partner, guides us into a deeper and more intimate relationship with ourselves, bringing light into the dark recesses of our psyches. Every now and then, the helping hand of someone who's had more experience of travelling in this territory can be very reassuring. For this reason, and to illuminate some of the realities of Tantra workshops and individual sessions, as well as to dispel some popular myths, I wish to give you a snapshot view of a little of what actually happens there.

TANTRA WORKSHOPS AND SESSIONS

You do not need to be young, beautiful or uninhibited to attend a Tantra workshop, nor do you need a partner. On the other hand, if you do come with a partner, you will remain with *your* partner, and your partner only, for the exercises and meditations presented. Tantric practitioners, or 'Tantrikas', come in all shapes, sizes, and ages, and from a wide range of backgrounds. They range from students, through newlyweds starting out on their journeys into sexual relating, to grandparents who have been married for over a generation and are looking for a new lease of life. James, a twenty-eight-year-old single professional, said at the end of his first Tantra weekend workshop that he felt as though he'd at last found a group of people and a way of being where he felt at home. Sean, a welder in his early fifties and his wife Jane, other participants at the workshop, said the same thing. Eleanor, a single mother of two teenagers, said that she felt like a soft and feminine, powerful and sexual woman for the first time in her life.

One of the key teachings in Tantra is about choice. In particular, it is about choosing appropriate boundaries for yourself in relation to another person. One of the first exercises we do at a workshop is about clearly and consciously communicating with a partner what level of contact you would like, at any given moment, from standing three feet apart to cuddling up close. Single people, who work with different partners for each exercise, in general choose more restrained boundaries than do couples, which is entirely appropriate and no less intimate than being part of a couple. I define intimacy ('into-me-see') as being honestly present in each moment, with clarity and integrity. Tantra is *not* all about throwing inhibition to the wind. It is about choosing which of our learned behaviours actually support our deepest longings, and which do not. It is about letting go of what no longer serves us, and strengthening what does. It's about giving our own, internal truth muscles a joyful workout.

> *I was extremely nervous about attending the Tantra course. I am a shy person by nature, and have never felt comfortable talking in a group of strangers. What motivated me to take the plunge (and I nearly turned back twice as I was driving there!) was a strong conviction that there must be more to life and sexual relationships than what I had, up till then, experienced. My fifteen years of marriage had ended eight years previously, and I still felt terribly alone and lacking in*

> *confidence. My ex-husband had been very domineering. Most of the time I had shied away from conflict and things went the way he wanted. I wanted to move on, to experience love and happiness, and to get back in touch with my libido again.*
>
> *As the workshop began, I found that I was really enjoying myself. The pace was very gentle and natural, and I felt much more relaxed than I ever would have imagined. Then it came to the exercise about choice and boundaries. I froze. In fact, the man who I was partnered with for the exercise looked friendly enough and was even quite attractive, but the thought of honestly telling him how close or distant I wanted him to be was terrifying. I don't think I'd ever been that direct in a relationship before. I had tended to think more about what the man wanted rather than what I wanted. I wasn't even sure if I knew what I wanted! I certainly didn't want him any closer than a foot away, and I told him so. He seemed strangely relieved. I realised then that he was almost as nervous as me. It was a very important moment for me, and I felt quite close to him as we stood there in silence together.*
>
> Margaret, 43, Care Worker

Moreover, to answer one of the most creatively asked questions, 'Um ... er ... do we have to, you know, um, take our clothes off?' the answer is no, not at the beginning. Later on, in more advanced workshops, the opportunity is given to remove clothing, if you choose to do so. It is always up to you.

Other fundamental aspects of Tantra workshops include reconnecting with the scope of our natural sensuality. Each person receives a delicate sensorial feast comprising a selection of sounds, smells, tastes, touch and sights, presented slowly and one at a time, to gently awaken and enliven each of the five senses. For most, this is an exceptionally moving experience of heightened sensitivity and enjoyment. The workshops also include movement meditations to facilitate the flow of sexual energy through the whole body, to promote health and well-being, as well as (when combined with sexual arousal, in the privacy of your own bedroom) to support the experience of whole-body orgasm. Traditional Tantric breathing practices are taught, for bringing you into contact with your 'chakras', the energy centres in the body, and for harmonising these within yourself and between you and a partner. In this way it is possible to experience sexuality that is also an expression of true love and a gateway to connecting with a wider sense of self. All of these practices are described in more detail later on in the book.

One couple, Felicia and Marcus, came to see me privately for some couples' sessions. Marcus was upset because Felicia frequently turned down his sexual advances, and now, as well as feeling horny and frustrated, he felt rejected and dejected. Felicia wanted sexual contact with Marcus, but didn't always want intercourse. She also felt that Marcus was too pushy, and often touched her in the wrong ways. Marcus was confused, and it seemed to him that he could never get it right.

Over the course of several sessions, I encouraged them to take turns in speaking and really listening to what the other wanted, and, more importantly, how they felt, without acting on any of it. From there, they took turns in asking for the quality of touch that they would like from each other, which turned out to be very different for each of them. Felicia preferred very, very fine touch. This helped her relax, to feel connected with Marcus, and to open up sexually. Marcus enjoyed strong, reassuring touch, as well as cuddles and spoken words. Receiving this helped him realise that Felicia did love and value him as a man. By establishing a firmer ground in communication, understanding and loving connectedness, they found that far more possibilities opened up for them sexually. Felicia was much more open than before to enjoying more raunchy sex, provided that she received some contact beforehand with Marcus that allowed her to feel in connection with him. She felt really turned on by Marcus's wildness and unrestrained passion, which was one of the things that had attracted her to him in the first place. Quite to his surprise, Marcus found that he actually enjoyed a subtler approach to lovemaking as well, and that he did not always have to ejaculate in order to feel fulfilled, as long as his inner 'caveman' could also have some space to play now and then.

Other reasons why people choose to do individual or couples' Tantra sessions may be to address specific issues such as fear of sex, recurring patterns in intimate relationships, or loss of love and libido. People also come to explore the wonders of Tantra in a setting where the attention is focused on their particular interests and explorations, for guidance in their practice and in how to bring these discoveries into everyday life.

Whatever your age, religion, profession or marital status, you can practise Tantra. Whether to heal, to enhance, to have fun, to transform, to try out, to let go or to meet God, these are all good reasons to give it a go. Whether no one but the goldfish ever knows that you've become a Tantrika (a Tantric practitioner), or whether you sing it out to the whole world, you now know a little of what to expect if you ever seek out support and tuition beyond the written word.

CHAPTER TWO

FIRST STEPS

The first thing you'll need to begin your adventures with Tantra is a little time to get started. As an important aspect of Tantra is about developing the taste for a slow and gentle build-up of energy that can infuse our whole being, rather than a more localised quick spurt of passion, I'd suggest that you approach this book in a similar manner. Take your time to really savour and integrate each stage of the journey before progressing to the next. This chapter introduces you to some delightful first steps that, like good wine, simply deepen and become even more delicious with age, experience and appropriate reverence.

This chapter focuses on making a 'Tantric date', and some of the components within it, summarised below:

1. Arrive fresh, prepared and ready to explore Tantra, at the time that you have pre-arranged your 'Tantric date'.
2. Prepare your 'sacred space', an atmosphere for Tantra (*see page 18*).

3. Greet yourself or your beloved with the gesture of namaste (*see page 25*).
4. Enjoy any of the meditations or exercises described in this book, beginning with Chapter 3 (if you are with a partner or like-minded friend) and Chapter 4 (if you are on your own). As you become more experienced, you can participate in the more advanced practices that are described throughout the book.
5. If you are with your beloved, depending on which meditation or exercise you have practised, the time you have, and how you both feel, you may choose to make love.
6. End with another namaste.
7. Take some time, either immediately or after a break, to share your experiences with your partner, or to write them down in a journal.

THE TANTRIC DATE

In my private practice, one of the first things that I generally suggest to many of my clients is that they initiate a Tantric date. About a third return the following session and tell me how and why that date didn't happen. It may sound like an obvious and ludicrously simple subject to give so much attention to, but in my experience it's the basic stumbling block for many newly toddling Tantrikas. So I'm going to give it lots of space, and hopefully by the end of this section, you'll find the topic as fascinating as I do.

What is a Tantric date?

You can either wait for a moment when you 'feel like it' or plan in advance to make a date for love. A Tantric date is a time when, as a single person or as a couple, you dedicate yourself to exploring Tantra. The best way to make the most of the meditations or exercises described from Chapter 3 onwards is to incorporate them into a

Tantric date. You may also wish simply to make love. Incorporating Tantra into lovemaking is covered in Chapter 6.

A Tantric date with your beloved self or partner has the following components:

1. A clear beginning time (agreed to by both partners).
2. A clear ending time (which can be extended by mutual agreement).
3. It is an alcohol and drug free zone. In order to preserve presence and clarity of mind and body, refrain from partaking of these substances for several hours before the date.
4. It is uninterrupted.
5. It has clear, shared intent.

Committing to a Tantric date has several advantages, but before I elucidate these, let me ask you a question. Why do you imagine that, while some of the highlights of television viewing are romance, love and even sex, most of us prefer to watch them on TV than to engage directly in the subject matter at home?

'I would if I had a partner,' you may say. Or 'I have a partner, but he/she isn't interested.' Perhaps you work long hours, and all you feel like doing when you get home is flopping out with a nice cold beer. Maybe you have young children, rebellious teenagers or elderly parents to take care of.

Undoubtedly the strains of modern life can be great, as we attempt to fulfil multiple roles, holding things together sometimes by a shoestring. Is it any surprise, then, that our personal relationships suffer, or that we feel out of touch with our own inner sense of fulfilment? If we forget to water the plants or feed and walk the dog, they will shrivel up and die. The water, food and exercise that a relationship requires to thrive may be more difficult to ascertain. The rewards, however, when we crack a code or solve a relationship riddle, can be awesome. It is up to us to make the commitment to finding out and implementing a self and relationship care programme.

Self-care

We do ourselves a disservice when we wait until we have a partner to be happy. Aside from anything else, this kind of attitude puts a lot of pressure on a relationship when one does materialise. If caring for ourselves, loving and listening to ourselves, is not familiar to us, we will expect our lover to care and listen to an extent that they may not be capable of, to satisfy that longing. Also, it will be difficult to fully receive love if we do not believe that we're lovable. These themes will be explored more fully later in the book. Besides, full and fulfilled individuals are far more attractive to potential new beloveds than inwardly empty and craving souls. So, solo Tantrikas, now's the time to set a date to celebrate yourself! Some excellent ways to get started on your own are given in Chapter 4.

Relationship care

Making time for your relationship is an essential first step towards paradise. There are many books available that focus on time management, such as *Take Time for Your Life* by Cheryl Richardson, and if this is a big theme in your life, I'd suggest exploring it further. At any rate, something special happens when you and your partner arrange a specific date to focus on each other. Something inside can go 'ahh', breathing a big sigh of relief. Simply by committing in this way to your relationship, things will start to improve. If all is already hunky-dory, they will get better still. So why wait; get out your diary and allocate some time to making a Tantric date!

How to make Tantric dates

Here are some keys to making an almost foolproof Tantric date with yourself or your beloved.

Key 1: start small

Begin by choosing a length and frequency of Tantric dates that's easily manageable for you, otherwise you're likely to default on your date. If you're trying to decide whether to arrange two-hour-long or one-and-a-half-hour-long dates, go for one and a half hours. Similarly, go for once a week if twice a week is optimistic. Then keep to what you've arranged, and you'll be rewarded with a sense of achievement and the beauty of the date itself.

Key 2: choose an optimum time of day

One of the reasons why intimate contact with a lover or with ourselves can fall short of its ultimate potential is simply that we've been programmed to think that evenings are the time for intimacy. Many of us are not at our best late at night, but are brimming with enthusiasm as the sun rises. In couples, it's not uncommon for early birds to be partnered with night owls, and in these cases you could consider perhaps a weekend late morning or afternoon. Find a time that works best for you.

Key 3: prepare for your date with 'transition time'

It would be unrealistic to expect that you can always, immediately and consistently, switch from being a hard-nosed, whirlwind 'to-do'-list machine, to expressing the passion and tenderness of the Tantric lover in you. It may take a while before 'mum', having entrusted her precious offspring to the babysitter, remembers that she's a sensual goddess. Let your date be sacred. Prepare for it by taking a walk, relaxing in a hot bath, listening to music or calling your best friend to debrief, so that you come fresh and in the moment to meet yourself or your partner. Remember to avoid drugs or alcohol, welcoming your mind and body au naturel.

Key 4: be clear that you will not be disturbed

Create a safe and secure container, a crucible, for your alchemical exploits. When your subconscious knows that this time is absolutely for you, that knowledge itself assists you in sinking more deeply into your truth. Switch off all phones. Do not answer the doorbell. If possible, make sure that your children are being looked after, ideally at some other location. If this is not realistic or appropriate, be clear about what you'll do if they knock at the door. Find some way of saying, clearly and unequivocally, 'Not now, later.' Then keep to your word.

Key 5: go ahead with the date, however you are feeling

Once you've made it there and the date begins, go for it! Don't cancel because you've got a headache or are in a bad mood. Acknowledge the headache or bad mood, and engage in your Tantric explorations in a way that is gentle and caring towards yourself, but doesn't let your ailment (which may also be resistance) run the show.

Given all I've said so far, I hope that this paragraph will be unnecessary. But just in case ... If, for any reason, you or your partner are late for the date, do postpone the 'discussion' about why and how this happened till afterwards. You may, of course, have an emotional response to your own or your partner's lateness (or to any other disruption to plans), and these emotions are valid. Experiment with acknowledging these feelings, letting them be here, and carrying on anyway. For a more detailed perspective on this, see pages 16 and 17.

Congratulations! If you're now luxuriating in a time and place set aside purely for you, the next step is to clarify and empower your intention for this date through creating 'sacred space'. You are then ready to embody the essence of Tantra with a traditional Tantric greeting called 'namaste'. After that we'll get going with some gentle and profound, delightful and eye-opening Tantric meditations, in Chapters 3 and 4. But first ...

Resistance

Quite possibly one of the first experiences you may have is of resistance. If this is the case, you may as well get to know your personal brand of resistance, as it is likely to be an ongoing companion in your Tantric journey.

Whether in partnership or as a single, at some point it is likely that you will meet with resistance to deepening in understanding and love of yourself and your beloved. Resistance is that part of you that is frightened of change. It prefers age-old beliefs and ways of doing things, even if they're not ultimately to your optimum advantage.

Resistance is clever and sneaky, and it can take some crafty detective work to sniff it out.

Sometimes resistance is open and honest, clear and concise. It is a feeling, a thought, a sense that says 'I don't want to do it. I'm frightened. I don't know what will happen.' More frequently, however, resistance takes on another disguise. Just before your Tantric date, you may become incredibly tired. This is a very special kind of tiredness. It's the sort connected with thoughts such as 'It's too much. I'm just too tired to do it today.' You feel completely pooped, even if ten minutes earlier you were bouncing around. It is a tense kind of tiredness, although you may not feel tense, and your mind becomes foggy and sluggish.

Alternatively, you may be late for your Tantric date. From what I hear from others, and from my own personal research (!), it seems that public transport knows when you're about to have a Tantric date and throws a spanner in the works. Road traffic, too, is significantly increased, and there is a far higher likelihood of a computer glitch or a sudden, urgent job to do at work. Your children will need you most just before a Tantric date, and you may receive long-distance phone calls from friends and relatives whom you have not spoken to for years. It can be an exciting time, this pre-date period! Look out, though; all of these occurrences can be undercover resistance!

These occurrences aren't always necessarily manifestations of resistance; your capacity to discern what is and isn't will grow over time. When you're extremely certain that you're not in resistance, and get emotionally highly charged at the suggestion that you might be, you probably are. To start with, it can be simpler just to assume that any reason for being late for a Tantric date is because of resistance.

This does not mean that you're wrong or bad for being in resistance. It's normal. Don't fight your resistance, just observe and get to know it. When we understand the wily ways of its wilful obstruction to our higher choices, we can skilfully avoid them. At its heart, resistance has your own interests in mind, as it sees them. Remember, it is the part of us that is afraid of change. When we develop compassion for our resistance, knowing where it comes from and what it's trying to do and why, it ceases to have power over us. Be patient and curious.

Why should we experience inner discord when committing to and moving towards what we truly desire and long for? It's quite a paradox. Old habits run deep. Perhaps as a child you longed for your mother's love and understanding, needed your father's attention and appreciation, and you didn't get it. Perhaps you came to believe that your needs, desires and longings were not important, and could never be fulfilled. This belief formed your identity. And now, maybe you're even afraid to believe that you might finally get what you always wanted but never had. To be open to receive what you've always wanted, you would need to risk not getting it, and once again feeling the pain of those previously unmet needs. Or, if your dreams came true, then where and who would you be? It would be completely unknown.

> *Ever since we started practising Tantra, Sandra had been the one to insist on making Tantric dates. She's far more organised than I am, it's true, but I'm the sort of man who likes to be spontaneous. I couldn't stand the rigidity of having to make love to order, according to some pre-arranged timetable. My idea of romance was to follow my urges whenever the mood took me, like having a quick fuck on the kitchen table after supper. But somewhere I knew that the Tantric path would bring me more pleasure, more joy, more juiciness than just carrying on as I had done before.*
>
> *Then, about a year ago, it stopped. It had been about two months and Sandra hadn't said a word about making a date. 'What's happening?' I asked her. She said she'd had enough of bending over backwards to arrange Tantric dates with me. She told me that it was like dragging a horse to water, and as far as she was concerned, she would rather go without Tantric intimacy than go through the whole unrewarding struggle. She announced that she had resigned from the job. I knew Sandra well enough to know that she meant it.*

It's funny how I felt an immense sense of freedom as she said that, and yet I also became aware of how much I valued our Tantric time together, and how much I missed relating to her in that way. 'I'll arrange some Tantric dates!' I offered. Sandra was both relieved and grateful, and for the first time, things went smoothly. From then on, everything changed. We had both moved away from trying to get each other to do things our own way, and paradoxically we both got what we wanted. I don't think it's anything we could have planned in advance. It's something that seemed to 'click' into place, when we were both completely fed up with how we had been interacting before.

LARRY, 57, COMPANY DIRECTOR

SACRED SPACE

Having arrived at your Tantric date, start by creating 'sacred space'. This means taking pleasure in preparing an inner and outer atmosphere conducive to practising Tantra. It can be as simple as taking a deep breath and remembering your motivations for exploring your inner landscape in this way, and beginning. Alternatively, you can take a bit more time relishing this process of inner and outer refurbishment.

Below are some ways in which you may like to create 'sacred space'. Do whatever feels right at the time, and feel free to add your own variations. You can take as long as half an hour or as little as five minutes.

Suggestion 1

Make sure that your physical surroundings are as conducive as possible to realising your intentions. You may like to hold the vision that whichever room you are using for Tantra will, for the duration of your date, become your 'Tantric Temple'. Some people prefer to use a room other than their bedroom for practising Tantra, to get away from associations with sleep, or less conscious sexual relating. Otherwise, your bedroom is a fabulous option.

Ideally, start with clearing any excess clutter in your surroundings. As you do so, let the process of clearing and tidying your physical space re-enforce your desire to devote your inner space, your attention, purely to yourself or to you and your partner.

Suggestion 2

You may like to first consider, then recite out loud, what qualities you would like to disengage from for the period of your Tantric date. You may already be aware of some of your own emotional and behaviour patterns that can tend to get in the way of realising your intentions. Some possibilities may be:

- My high expectations of myself and others.

- Having preconceived ideas of what the outcome of a certain meditation or exercise should be.

- My tendency to 'be in my head', thinking about the past and future, fantasising, and so on.

- Fear of being hurt.

- Fear of not being good enough.

- Shame about enjoying my body.

- Resentment towards my partner from the past.

- 'It'll never make any difference anyway, so what's the point?'

Creating sacred space is about remembering ways in which you've habitually tripped yourself up in the past, and choosing to do it differently this time.

You can use phrases such as, 'I, Leora, choose to let go of shame about my body.' If you like, these words can be accompanied and re-enforced by cleansing gestures such as ringing bells, beating drums or burning cleansing herbs such as sage. Including your name personalises the statement and can make it more powerful! Another option is to write down what you choose to disengage from on a piece of paper, put it in a dustbin and leave the bin outside the room. Any aspects you wish to pick up again afterwards, you can. The rest you can dispose of as you see fit.

Suggestion 3

If it appeals to you, you may like to beautify your temple, making it sensual and romantic. You can:

- Light candles.
- Burn incense or essential oils.
- Arrange fresh flowers.

Khalil Gibran, in his mystical book *The Prophet*, says, 'Where shall you seek beauty, and how shall you find her unless she herself be your way and your guide?' As we recognise the importance of beauty in our outer and inner worlds, we create more of it, and become more deeply immersed in it. We come to live more beautiful lives.

Suggestion 4

Sit or stand comfortably in your temple. Take a moment to appreciate where you are. Connect with your intentions for this date.

Be as specific as you can, and try to keep your intentions focused on yourself. If you would like your partner to open up more to you, perhaps your intention could be to discover, through attention and deep listening, what it is that you do that results in your partner either opening up or closing down, and why. Other sorts of intentions may be to:

- Stay as present as possible in each moment.
- Remember to relax and breathe deeply.
- Be open to spontaneity.
- Be as open to your partner as you are able to be.
- Be gentle with yourself.
- Let go of expectations.
- Embrace your sexuality in all its aspects.
- Know the god/goddess in you.
- Have as much fun as possible.

Recite, write, whisper or sing your intentions, for example, 'I, Leora, choose to let go of preconceptions and to be open to whatever happens in each moment!' Let the words be your own. I like to use the word 'choose', since words such as 'hope' and 'wish' are hypothetical, and 'want' is in the future. If you are with a partner, it's particularly powerful and intimate to sit opposite each other, hold hands, maintain eye contact and breathe together for a short while in silence. Then speak your intentions to each other.

Suggestion 5

If there's anyone who you consider to be a mentor, a wise person, a teacher or a master, you can invite their support and presence to guide and care for you during this time. These people can include those you know personally like your grandmother or a special friend, those you know about such as Mother Meera or the Dalai Lama, and mythical, religious and spiritual beings too, such as the Buddha, Jesus Christ, Archangel Gabriel, Shekhinah, Pan or Venus Aphrodite.

Having prepared your sacred space, you are now ready to greet yourself and your partner with a namaste.

NAMASTE

The word 'namaste' in Sanskrit and Hindi translates simply as 'greeting'. However its symbolic meaning goes far deeper. In fact, it is simultaneously an excellent technique for self-reflection and a profound meditation on unity.

On an interpersonal level, namaste means: 'I honour you as a mirror of myself' – a simple phrase to say, but of vast significance if you really mean it! In a relationship, honouring your partner as a mirror means really taking responsibility for what this person, by simply being who they are, is showing you about you. This can happen in several ways.

In the most straightforward sense, when you honour another as a mirror of yourself, you notice what qualities and character traits you see in them, and how you respond and react to these perceptions. So if you meet a confident person and shrink to become a meek and obsequious jellyfish, you can see them as mirroring to you a lost part of yourself. You can then begin to investigate what happened to your own confidence and self-esteem, and from there, how you might reintegrate that part of your being. Conversely, if you meet a person who is less open than yourself, perhaps who even speaks untruthfully at times, and you notice yourself feeling angry or superior and judging them, you might take this opportunity to develop a little compassion. You could ask yourself if there are any circumstances when you have put on a brave face or brittle exterior, when you have hidden or obscured the truth, perhaps to hide a crying or ashamed child underneath. Your perception of this other person, this 'mirror', would no longer be the same.

Another facet to seeing someone as a mirror of yourself is to recognise what aspects of yourself arise in this relationship. In my case, I married a man who has a very flexible relationship with time. In other words, he was (and this is more rarely the case now) frequently late – late for dates, late home from nights out with the boys and especially late for Tantra workshops! This used to drive me completely and utterly nuts, and I would become a nervous wreck when he was even five minutes behind schedule. All I wanted at those moments was to send him back to the shop and get a new, improved husband with an inbuilt timer!

Gradually and rather reluctantly, through hearing myself say it enough times to others, I considered the possibility of seeing my husband as a mirror. What I saw, as I looked at my reflection, was that I felt both extremely anxious and completely powerless when someone I depended on was late. I realised that this stemmed from when I was a child, and my mother, who I relied upon for many things, including transport to and from school, birthday parties and other important occasions, was almost never on time. I suffered the consequences of chastisement at school and insecurity socially as a result, and yet I was unable to effect any change on my mother's behaviour. In reconnecting with this memory I was able to share my more vulnerable feelings on this subject, without blame, with my husband. I was also able to work on healing this unresolved issue in myself, and to realise that as an adult, I was now in charge and could take action to prevent myself being 'left in the lurch'.

When we're truly able and willing to see another human being as a mirror, both comfortable and uncomfortable meetings can ultimately become gifts.

In its ultimate expression, namaste represents the unity of all things – that essential oneness of Spirit, God, the Universe and Truth that is beyond duality. On this level, namaste means: 'I honour the Divine Essence in you.' Another, more poetic way to express this is: 'I honour that place in you where the whole Universe resides. When I am in that place in me, and you are in that place in you, there is just one of us.' It is about looking more deeply than the level of personality to that essential humanness, that essential existence, where we are all the same.

'Looking' in this way requires more than eyes and understanding. It takes heart. Namaste can also be called the 'heart salutation'. Becoming more in touch with your heart is a large part of what this book is about.

If you're by yourself, you can literally greet the reflection of yourself in the mirror. Whether you're in an ongoing sexual-loving relationship or not, I recommend greeting yourself in the mirror with a namaste. Your feelings and beliefs about yourself will be very apparent as you do this, and it's an incredible springboard to developing a more compassionate relationship with yourself, and ultimately to remembering the beauty of who you really are.

The gesture

Finally, on a practical level, namaste is a gesture that, in Tantra, signifies the beginning and end of a Tantric 'date', or of any kind of intimate meeting with yourself or another person. It's a way of entering into inner sacred space, and then of expressing gratitude for what we have learned, experienced or enjoyed in that time.

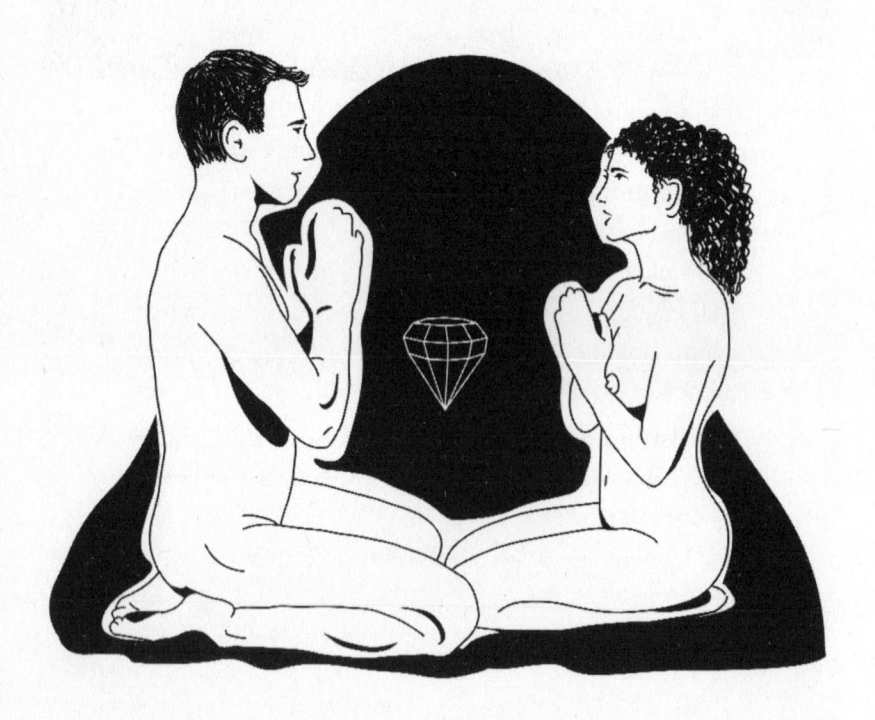

BREATHING IN, BRING YOUR HANDS TOGETHER IN FRONT OF YOUR HEART

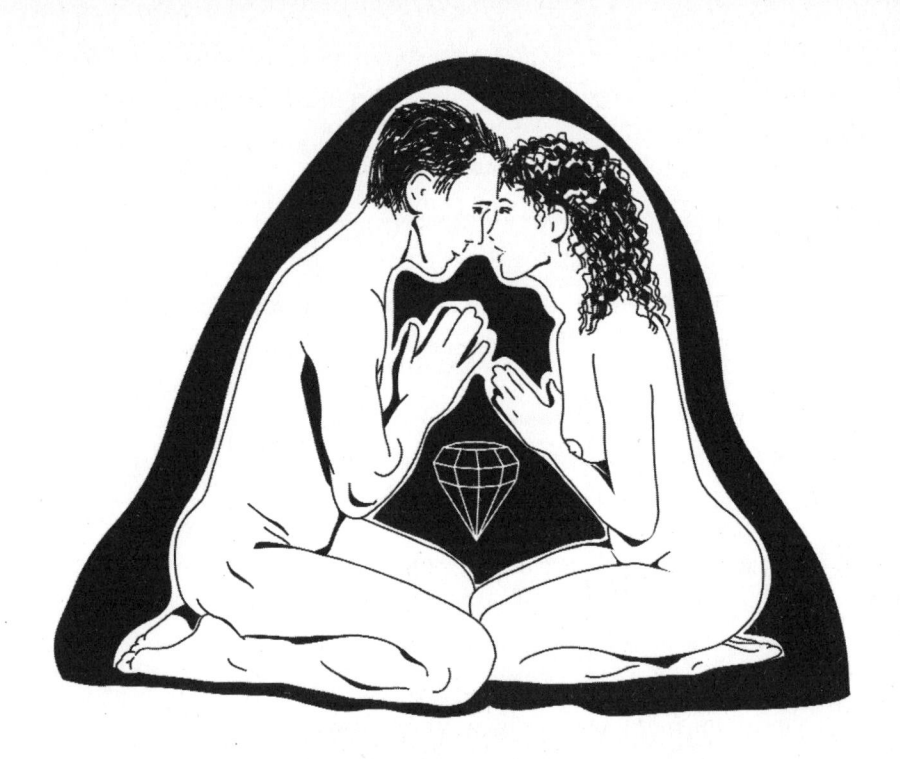

TOUCH FOREHEADS WITH YOUR PARTNER

The Technique

The gesture of namaste, described below, is very simple.

- Begin by sitting or standing facing your partner, or your own reflection in the mirror if you are on your own. (By the way, the gesture of namaste can be shared with anyone, not only your life or sexual partner. Try it also with interested friends and relatives.)

- Take a few moments just to 'arrive' with each other, coming into eye contact in silence. Then let your arms hang loose and relaxed, apart and pointing towards the earth. You can imagine

First steps — 25

that as you begin the namaste, you are drawing up the energy of the earth (life force, embodiment, solidity and ground) into your heart. You can imagine that you're holding the precious jewel of love in your hands.

- Together (just sense the right moment), inhale and bring the hands together in front of the heart. See the illustration on page 24.

- Exhaling, and with a straight back, bend forwards from the hips and, keeping your eyes open, let your forehead touch that of your partner. See the illustration on page 25. As you bend forwards towards each other, your love travels up to your 'third eye' – the mystical eye between the eyebrows, the eye that looks inwards. This is your centre of inner vision, insight, clarity and bliss. As you touch foreheads, you meet from this place of clarity, symbolising your intention for a conscious and mutually life-enhancing exchange.

- Inhale again, straightening your back, and return to the 'prayer position' with your hands in front of your heart. While straightening up, your focus returns to your heart, acknowledging any gratitude you feel for this meeting.

- Relax your arms as you exhale, returning your hands to their original positions pointing towards the earth. As you release your arms again, you 'ground' the experience of this meeting, returning your attention once more to the earth.

- Then, still in eye contact, either simultaneously or sequentially, say the word 'namaste'.

Once you have got used to this quite intimate gesture, which may initially seem a little strange or foreign, you will no longer need to think about whether you're 'doing it right', and you can enter into the spirit of the gesture. You may lightly ask yourself what this person you're greeting is mirroring to you. When you've got the sense of how each meeting contains the seeds of growth for you, let go of looking for a mirror. Allow yourself to just receive the essence of this person through their eyes (*see* also 'eye gazing', *page 64*). Remember that as human beings we all hurt sometimes, and what we all truly want is to love and be loved.

CONTINUING AND COMPLETING YOUR DATE

Having set and arrived at a Tantric date, with yourself or with your partner, created a sacred space and shared the greeting of namaste, you can continue to dive into any of the exercises or meditations that follow. Those in Chapter 3 are ideal if you are with a partner; those in Chapter 4 are perfect if you are on your own. Remember, even if you are in a loving relationship, don't skip spending some time alone, as this is invaluable to developing your own sense of self-love and energetic flow within your body. If you are a couple, you can either progress to making love, or you may choose not to. End your date with a namaste and take time to share or write down your experiences.

CHAPTER THREE

(DELICIOUS BEGINNINGS FOR COUPLES)

This chapter offers three short, delightful and straightforward ways to enjoy bringing your sensuality, love and spirit into contact with another person, plus a more in-depth ritual to awaken the senses. You can enjoy all of these 'Tantric tasters' with a good friend, who need not be your sexual partner. All can be fully appreciated while remaining fully clothed. If you are with an intimate partner, you may also sample them naked.

MELTING HUG

And when [love's] wings enfold you, yield to him …
KHALIL GIBRAN, *THE PROPHET*

A melting hug is a beautiful way to connect simply and deeply with another person. It is about sharing, and more importantly receiving, meaningful human contact. A melting hug offers us the opportunity to let down our brittle defences and enjoy our own softness and tenderness, as well as the softness and tenderness of another. Melting hugs can be shared with anyone, friends (of the same and other sex), family or your lover. A melting hug may mean different things to different people at different times. The defining feature of a melting hug is two people truly arriving together in a simple embrace, without agenda, through being fully present in each moment. It's called a 'melting hug' because as you remain together, breathing and relaxing, receiving each other through this contact, the boundaries between the two of you can start to melt away, and some merging of 'me' with 'you' can happen.

More than once, I've been told by a workshop participant that 'Having sex is easy for me. But hugging is really scary!' The melting hug

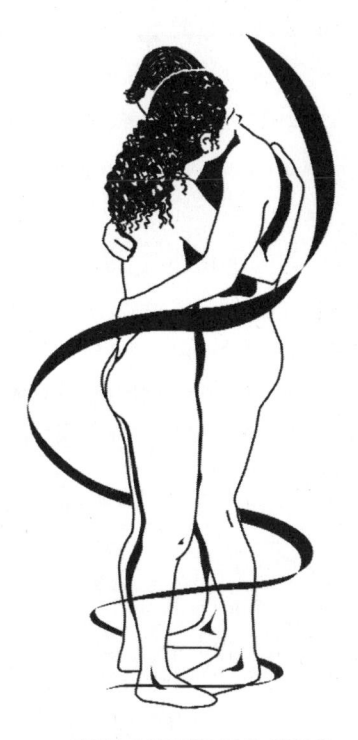

THE MELTING HUG

Delicious beginnings for couples — 29

is about intimacy rather than eroticism. At the right time and with the right person, it may also have a strong sensual or sexual component. The main point, however, is not whether you are aroused or not, it's about enjoying being with this person in this moment, and not trying to do or get anything else.

The Technique

This is how to share a melting hug:

- The melting hug starts as you and your partner face, see, notice and sense one another. It is possible that spontaneous smiles may radiate from your or your partner's face, or sometimes even tears of joy or release. There is, however, no right or wrong way to feel.

- It is advisable to continue breathing at all times. Holding the breath means obstructing the natural flow of feelings and energy, and this is a time to let it all hang out.

- Move gently towards each other, opening your arms and your hearts.

- Come into soft, relaxed full-body contact, and let your arms naturally enfold each other. Generally, one arm goes over, and the other under the arms of your partner. This allows for a comfortable and snug fit. For huggers of different heights, either the taller partner can stand comfortably with legs astride (so that he stands at the height of the shorter partner), or the shorter partner can stand on a book, a step or a small stool.

- Your arms and hands remain still, without patting or stroking; your bodies are in contact, just resting, being, feeling the connection.

- Both of you breathe in harmony, inhaling and exhaling together. Your eyes are closed, and your attention is with the rise and fall of the breath, and the warm sensations and the feelings generated by the physical and energetic contact.

- A melting hug can last from thirty seconds to fifteen minutes or more.

- You can enjoy a melting hug standing up, sitting or lying down (where it becomes a 'melting cuddle').

I have been nervous about touch all my life. In my family, no one was ever demonstrative, and I always felt quite awkward at family gatherings or other occasions where someone tried to kiss or hug me. I generally pulled away, kind of by reflex. The thing is, that wasn't what I really wanted underneath it all. It's just that I didn't know how to respond to touch, and felt extremely embarrassed.

It was so liberating to be in an environment where I could start again. I didn't have to do anything that I didn't want to do, but I didn't have to stay isolated either. At first I couldn't really 'melt' into a melting hug, but after a while I learned to relax enough to really enjoy it. Actually, I think I'm quite a tactile person, but I never admitted it to myself before, because I found touch so scary.

I think it'll make a big difference in my life in lots of ways. Especially with men. I hope now that I know the difference between affection and sex, I won't be so drawn to sleeping with someone to get affection.

LISA, 32, ESTATE AGENT

BACK-TO-BACK DANCE

The back-to-back dance is a fun way to awaken your natural, innocent, whole-body sensuality. It can be done with your beloved, or with a like-minded friend. Because it is *your* sensuality that is being awakened, feeling sensual does not need to be *about* the other person. It is something of you that you choose to enjoy and share, and it need not *mean* anything more than that.

Back-to-back dance, part 1

The initial focus of awareness in the dance is on your relationship with your own body. For many people, this simple and innocent focus on sensuality for its own sake, without an agenda, can be truly liberating. Often we shut away our natural exuberance and sexiness for fear of others' or our own judgements, or of adverse consequences. We may have, in the past, felt that we had to 'perform' sexually, without taking adequate notice of our own enjoyment of our body, and how to contact that. Now, as you shed the need to be anyone or any way other than who and how you actually are, and you give yourself permission and encouragement to succumb to sensuality, you are initiating a new love affair with you.

It is also common, however, for some people to feel anything but sensual in response to the invitation to engage with the pleasures of their pelvises in this way. This can be the case particularly if you have suffered any kind of sexual trauma that has not yet been healed, or if you grew up in an environment where sensuality and sexuality were frowned upon or scorned. A phrase well worth remembering is that 'Love brings up everything other than itself'. So don't be surprised if, as you lovingly attempt to bring your awareness to the area of your body around your genitals, what you experience is everything in you that obscures your natural, innocent free sensual expression.

This is a necessary stage in the process of healing and reclaiming your sensuality and sexuality, so don't be perturbed. If the feelings of discomfort are very strong, I'd recommend ending the back-to-back dance for now and spending some time writing down your experiences, or talking about them with your partner. Return to the back-to-back dance as soon as you are able to do so. Repeat the 'pause and write' procedure should you need to.

> ### The Technique
>
> You will need ten to fifteen minutes in total and some earthy music. A steady drumbeat and didgeridoos are a good combination. Specific music suggestions are given in the resources section (*see page 250*).
>
> Start by greeting each other, looking in the mirror of each other's eyes and acknowledging the essence, the divine, the god or goddess in each other with a namaste.
>
> - Put on the music, and stand back to back with your partner with your eyes closed.
>
> - As you breathe, become aware of the sensations and qualities of the physical contact between you. Do you feel a pleasant warmth? Is your partner's back rigid or relaxed? Are you stiffening your muscles, or are you gently resting your weight on your partner? Do you miss having eye contact? Do you feel a sense of togetherness?
>
> - Imagine that you are meeting each other for the first time, getting to know one another, and communicating non-verbally, simply through your backs. What are you saying to each other? What would you like to communicate?
>
> - Now bring your attention to your pelvis. Notice how you feel as you contact the sensations in your genitals, pelvic floor, bottom and hips from the inside. What is it like for you to feel into your pelvis? What, up till now, has been the quality of your relationship with your own genital region? How would you like this relationship to be? Remember that you have the

> power to choose to relate to any part of yourself with loving respect, starting from now.
>
> - As you hear the music, let your pelvis begin to respond. Move and rotate your hips, letting your pelvis wake up and stretch. As you move, take some delicious deep breaths, perhaps exhaling with a sigh or a sound.
>
> - Welcome the sensuality in your pelvis. Find the fun and playful spontaneity, the joy and sensuality in your pelvis dance. Celebrate, through this movement, breath and sound, that you *are* a sensual man or woman.
>
> - Notice any sensations, feelings or recurrent thoughts that arise as you do this.

Back-to-back dance, part 2: meeting your partner

So, here you are, moving your pelvis, either suffused with satisfying sensuality, or tasting tantalising titbits of pleasure while welcoming with awareness your learned reactions to sensual expression. Now it's time to notice that your pelvis is not alone!

> ### The Technique
>
> Carry on with the back-to-back dance, acknowledging your feelings, and yet still returning your attention to the physical sensations in your pelvis in the here and now.
>
> - Become aware that right in contact with you is another playful pelvis which can't wait to get to know yours. Imagine your pelvises to be two sensual snakes introducing themselves and getting to know each other. Let them dance and sway together.

- As your sensual, snake-like pelvises continue their dance, imagine that these two snakes are so thrilled with meeting each other and moving together, that they extend their presence and their dance into your backs and spines. Let the whole of your spine become a serpent-like sensual organ. Stretch and undulate together, responding to each other's movements.

- After a few minutes, or when the music ends, let your dance together find a natural conclusion, and once more just rest, standing together back to back, perhaps gently swaying.

- Notice any sensations or feelings in your body, any thoughts in your head.

- Gently step out of physical contact, turn around, open your eyes and come into eye contact. Again notice what sensations, feelings or thoughts are present for you at this moment.

- Find a way to thank and acknowledge each other without words (a melting hug, perhaps, or simply holding hands and smiling), and then complete this dance with a namaste.

- Take a few minutes to share in words what this meeting was like for you, and what you discovered.

FINGERTIP HEART DANCE

One of my teachers once told me that 'to connect sex and love is one of the most difficult things for a human being to do'. I had not appreciated this before, but when he said it, it made complete sense. And, essentially, connecting love and sex is a large part of what Tantra is about.

What's the challenge? It's about discovering and choosing the strength in vulnerability. To experience the joy and bliss of truly making love we need to drop our masks, letting our innermost being show its naked brilliance.

The fingertip heart dance can help us to do this. It is a way of cutting the crap and getting straight to the heart of the matter. It's a great one for dissolving hard-and-fast post-argument entrenchments, and for opening up a romantic, tender erotic flow.

> ### *The Technique*
>
> The exercise takes only ten to fifteen minutes. Some slow, heartful music is helpful (*see* Resources, *page 250*, for suggestions).
>
> - Start with a namaste.
>
> - Turn on the music. Stand opposite each other and hold your hands out in front of you so that you touch each other's fingertips.
>
> - Then close your eyes.
>
> - As you breathe, imagine that you're breathing in and out of your heart. You may visualise, feel sense or just know that by intending or imagining your heart breathing, you will become more in touch with your heart centre.
>
> - Let your chest fill with air as you inhale, and simply relax as you exhale. How is your heart at this moment?
>
> - You may receive an image, such as a big, red vibrant heart glowing with love (or a heart surrounded by brick walls), for example, or you may have a physical sensation such as warmth or tightness in your chest area. Alternatively you may have a feeling, such as love, sadness, numbness or exhilaration.
>
> - You don't need to be at all sure what's going on in your heart, as you may not have ever connected with your heart in this way

before. Just be curious. See this as an opportunity to relate to this essential part of yourself, to your feelings more than to your thoughts.

- Imagine or intend that whatever love is in your heart is expanding so that it extends out from your chest and into both of your shoulders, arms, hands and fingertips.

- There is definitely some love flowing through your heart, otherwise you wouldn't be alive, and as you imagine it flowing out and into your arms, you may find that there's more available than you thought at first! Your arms and hands are natural extensions of your heart; they're vessels through which your love expresses itself in the world. So as you stand here, eyes closed, fingertips to fingertips, you're also standing heart to heart.

- Bring your awareness now into the contact between your fingertips and those of your partner, and simultaneously become aware of contact between your heart and theirs.

- As you breathe, notice the feelings or sensations that this meeting evokes in you. Then, through the medium of your fingertips, let your heart express its feelings, its hopes and its longings with a movement, a gesture, a dance, keeping your fingertips in contact with your partner's. Remember that you can't get it wrong (or right!), so there's no point in trying. Just loosen up and let your dance be as it is.

- It may seem a little awkward at first, but as you continue you'll find that your heart is moving your fingertips without you having to think or do anything. Simply stay curious and open to the dance of your heart, and the dance of your two hearts together.

- Still touching at the fingertips, let your heart's dance include the whole of your arms and upper torso, so that the movement originates, physically as well as energetically, from your chest. Welcome whatever feelings come.

- Now's the time to include your sexuality and sensuality. Imagine your love trickling or cascading from your heart down your torso and into your pelvis and genitals, filling them with loving aliveness. Let your pelvis move.

- Experiment with oscillating, rotating, rocking or gently vibrating motions in your hips, and see which motions feel most enjoyable and genuine for you. When you're in contact with your sexiness or gentle sensuality, bring your awareness back to your heart and fingertips, continuing to move your pelvis. In this way, your love awakens your sexuality, and your sexuality and passion express themselves through your heart and your fingertips. It's a two-way flow.

- Look for a softness, a receptivity in your dance, rather than a 'doingness'. Notice how that current flows within you, and between you and your beloved.

- When your dance finds its natural conclusion, or when the music ends, rest a while in fingertip contact in stillness, noticing where you've arrived at with each other and in yourself.

- Then slowly and consciously move your fingertips apart, keeping your attention on the ongoing connection between the two of you.

- Open your eyes, receiving your beloved with your gaze, then thank and acknowledge what has passed between you with a namaste.

- Take a few minutes to share your experiences.

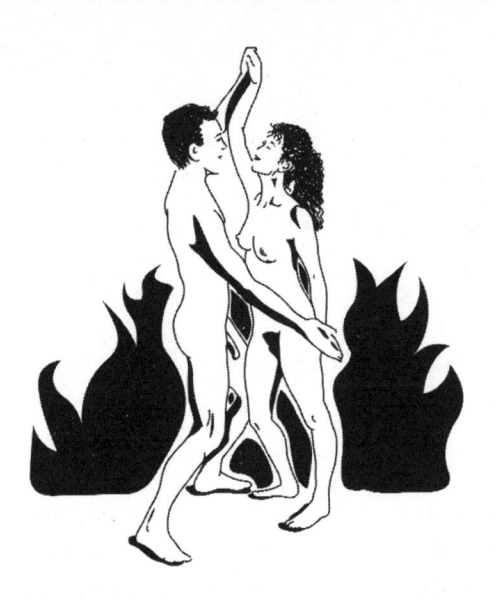

THE FINGERTIP HEART DANCE

In another, very beautiful variation of the fingertip heart dance, open your eyes as you start to move. Keep your eyes open, receiving your partner with your eyes throughout the dance. If you need to close them at any time to reconnect with yourself, then do so. Many people find that the 'eyes open' fingertip dance is more personal and intimate, while the 'eyes closed' version is more transpersonal and expansive. You'll find out for yourself what is true for you, and that is what counts!

> *Colin's sex drive was higher than mine and this was creating problems, so we went for some couples' sessions with Leora. At our second session, she introduced us to the 'fingertip heart dance'. I thought that Colin would think that it was naff, but actually it was quite the opposite. He loved it, and when we opened our eyes I could see that he was close to tears. This was the starting point for us of a long discussion about love and sex. The bottom line was that I came to see that it wasn't that I didn't want sex per se; I just wanted to know that I was loved as well. And it turned out that part of Colin's constant desire for sex was also about*

> *wanting love. We both recognised our own individual difficulties in combining sex and love, and have been able to work on these. In the process we are becoming much closer, and now when we do have sex it's mostly very loving.*
>
> PATRICIA, 47, MANAGER

SENSORY AWAKENING RITUAL

When eating or drinking, become the taste of the food or drink and be filled.

SHIVA SUTRA

Tantra sees the senses as gateways to Spirit. It is through being totally absorbed in sensory experience that the discursive mind can drop away and we 'become' the sound, smell, taste, touch or sight. In this moment we transcend the ordinary boundaries of self and other and so move from separate, dualistic perception into oneness and wholeness.

The sensory awakening ritual offers an exquisite opportunity for this absorption to occur. By receiving delicate sensory delights with each of the five senses, one at a time, slowly, sensitively and spaciously, only the strongest of resolves could prevent you from being in some way touched by the experience.

The ritual is offered as a gift by one lover to their beloved, and requires preparation, which could involve some shopping. You can either both give and receive a sensory awakening on the same occasion, or spread out the giving and receiving over two dates. Either way, leave plenty of time, as this experience cannot be rushed. Preparation can take anything from twenty minutes to one hour or more, some of which can be done well in advance of the date. The ritual itself takes thirty minutes to one and a half hours, depending on how you choose to conduct it.

Preparation

Gather a few or several sensory stimuli from each of the five sensory modalities. Some suggestions are given below. Choose a minimum of three items from each list. Also find something (like a scarf) that can be used as a blindfold.

> **Sound** Bells, a wind chime, a rattle, drums, a whistle or flute, any other musical instrument that you can play, beautiful pieces of recorded music without words, your own beautiful voice.
>
> **Smell** Scented flowers, perfume, essential oils, herbs, pleasant-smelling food, aromatic fruits, scented areas of your anatomy.
>
> **Taste** Fresh fruits (including unusual or exotic ones if possible), something savoury (nuts, crisps, fresh bread), chocolate, a refreshing soft drink.
>
> **Touch** A feather, something furry, a silk scarf, a cuddly toy.
>
> **Sight** Candles and night lights, candlesticks and night light holders, a special cloth (but don't be heartbroken if some wax spills on it), beautiful statues, crystals, evocative and meaningful pictures, sea shells, jewellery, fresh fruits and flowers. Alternatively, simply your own beautiful face.

Do your preparations in private. Do not let your partner see what you are doing. Cut up the food to be tasted into small, bite-sized pieces and arrange them decoratively on plates. Prepare more food than you need for the ritual (only one taste of each), so that there will be some left over. Select a room to become your temple, and make sure that it's warm. Clear away any clutter and prepare a sumptuous seat for your beloved. In front of the seat, leaving space for them to stretch out if they choose to do so, create a beautiful altar. Arrange everything – the musical items, scents, foods, touchy-feely things and objects of beauty – in an artful way, interspersed with candles and night lights. Imagine how it will look with the lights out, illuminated only by candlelight.

Prepare your body lovingly. You will be the priest or priestess of this temple of the senses. Dress in something simple and sensual. Ask your partner to wear minimal clothing. They may be naked if they like.

The Technique

Allow thirty to ninety minutes for the ritual, and start off in a room other than your temple.

The first steps

- Begin with a namaste.

- Remind your partner that this is a time when you will be devoted to them. If they need anything (a glass of water, to use the bathroom, a tissue, etc.), they should remain blindfolded and ask you to assist them.

- Let them know that they will soon be guided into a temple of the senses, and that they will be enjoying simple gifts from each sensual modality, one at a time. Invite them to relax and enjoy!

- They should refrain from speaking (other, non-verbal sounds are welcome) for the duration of the ritual, aside from asking for anything they need.

- Blindfold your beloved and lead them slowly and carefully into the temple, assisting them to recline on their sacred throne.

- Throughout the whole ritual, be slow and gentle, sensitive and kind. Support your partner in trusting you and letting go. Do not talk to your partner unless you sense that they are nervous and would benefit from some reassurance. If you sense that they are at all confused or uncomfortable, ask them how they are and if there's anything they need.

Sound

- Begin with sound.

- If you don't have any of the 'raw' musical items listed, it's fine to use recorded music for this whole section. In that case choose a variation of recorded music, from spacey to funky to gooey.

- Start with a soft sound like that of a small bell. Ring the bell (or produce whatever sound you're making) some distance away from your partner, then ring it again closer. Experiment with space, distance, movement and volume of sound. Bear in mind, however, that your partner is in a sensitised state, so don't make any sudden, nearby loud sounds, which may shock them.

- Move on to other instruments, like rattles and drums, creating a gentle crescendo. You can also play with vocal sounds such as laughter, animal sounds, humming and singing.

- Finish with a romantic or moving piece of recorded music, or sing a love song.

Scent

- Pause. Then start with the smells.

- Offer your beloved one smell at a time. Position each flower under the nose of your partner, giving them time to sniff two or three times. Pause before offering another smell.

- When presenting essential oils and perfumes, waft them in the air a little distance away from your beloved's nostrils, then slowly come closer.

- You may also include the natural scents of your own body.

Taste

- Follow on with taste.

- Feed your partner a piece of fruit. Let them savour the flavour slowly. Wait a while, then offer them something different.

- For extra fun and sensuality, stroke your partner's lips with the fruit before sliding it into their mouth.

- It's amazing how flavour and texture come to life when you are devoting such exquisite attention to eating. It can be the gustatory equivalent of hearing an orchestral masterpiece when previously you'd been listening to an amateur cellist.

- Being fed in this way requires a degree of trust and receptivity that may not be familiar to you or your partner. Bear in mind that this sweet and playful ritual can evoke strong feelings for people who, in the past, have suffered breaches of trust. The feeding stage specifically has the potential to summon up body memories (both pleasant and unpleasant) of being fed as a baby. This stage may be particularly challenging for those who have suffered oral sexual abuse. Always ask how your partner is feeling if they look in any way distressed, and never force-feed them.

- Replacing old memories of trauma with new, loving and enjoyable experiences can be extremely healing, if approached sensitively. Most importantly, the recipient needs to know that right here and now, *they* are in charge (it's about *their* delight and sensory awakening. You are their devotee). You can remind them that they may say 'no' whenever they like, and modify the ritual to support what they need at the time (*see also page 40*). For example, if your beloved is jumpy about being fed, you can place the items of food in their hand (one at a time!) and invite them to feed themselves.

Touch

- Work on touch next.

- Begin with a feather. Very, very slowly, and very softly, caress the skin of your beloved, starting with an extremity such as their hand or foot. Progress in a continuous movement up their arm or leg, stroking over their torso and concluding with their face. (The subject of delicate 'Tantric touch' is covered more fully in Chapter 11.)

- Next offer the same quality of light, slow, sensitive, continuous touch with your fingertips, in a similar fashion.

- For a grand finale you can gently stroke your partner with silks, furs, your hair, breasts, lips or whatever takes your fancy, keeping the contact soft, light and moving from the extremities to the torso and face.

- Cuddly toys are ideal for evoking the playful inner child in your beloved. Bring the toy to life, as it nuzzles, kisses and plays with them!

Sight

- You have two options for how you engage with the final stage, that of sight.

- *Option 1* If you have prepared a beautiful altar, now's the time to light the candles and night lights. Check that everything is arranged beautifully. Then you may either invite your partner to remove their blindfold when they are ready, or you can do it for them. Sit back and let them feast their eyes on the gorgeous temple that you have created for them. Let them receive the sight, which will be vastly more fresh and vibrant after their time in sensory meditation, and having been deprived of sight for this period.

- *Option 2* Alternatively, you yourself and the god or goddess within you become the altar. Sit in front of your partner, eyes open and with a receptive gaze (for more on receptive gaze, see page 62). Again either they or you remove their blindfold.

Sit in silence, and let your beloved drink in the sight of you. Let them receive your physical beauty, and more importantly, the love, beauty and wonder that is your true nature.

Conclusion

- You may like to hug or embrace.
- Share a namaste, then take some time to offer thanks and appreciations, and to talk about your experience of the sensory awakening ritual.

Below is Alison's account of her first experience of this ritual.

Blindfolded and guided to sit on a cushion, I was a little apprehensive at first. My everyday, busy mind relaxed, loosened its control and allowed my senses to awaken. Without warning I entered into a state of sensual delight, utterly absorbed in the sounds, tastes and textures, enticing me to surrender to each new experience as it arose. The outside dropped away, and I sank into an inner space of womb-like intimacy.

The final part of the ritual was, for me, the most powerful. A secret altar had been created, and as I removed my blindfold, my eyes were dazzled by the bright glow of candlelight. I stood in awe of the beauty and sacredness in front of me, bathed in a warm sea of bliss. It was an unforgettable experience.

ALISON, 33, MOTHER

CHAPTER FOUR

TANTRA ALONE AND AS A SINGLE PERSON

Tantric teachings offer us a vision of relationships where a man and a woman come together like a king and a queen. The king and queen are both full and whole in themselves, joining with each other as a celebration of themselves, and to create even more joy, bliss and ecstasy. (If you are in a homosexual partnership you may like to think about the union of the king in each of you with the queen in the other, and vice versa.) Most of us, however, enter into relationships more like beggars, desperately longing for our beloved, who we see as the fountain of love, to make us whole. Many romantic pop songs, novels and films reinforce this belief that we are incomplete without our 'other half'. The problem is that our other half is expecting the same from us. 'Give me love!' we demand. 'OK, but you give me love first!' our partner responds. We've reached a stalemate, a sense of poverty where there isn't enough love to go around.

Of course, this doesn't happen straight away. To begin with, both partners do actually become fountains of love, treasure troves bearing gifts that they didn't even know they possessed. And then, sooner or later, after months or years, it starts to slowly fade, or else to dramatically crumble before our eyes.

Tantra takes us by the hand in these moments of descending darkness and says, 'Don't lose hope! There is a stairway back to heaven. But you'll need to build it, brick by brick, inside yourself.' It shows us ways to develop our inner masculine and feminine selves, to nourish the king and queen within, to find wholeness within ourselves. The good news is that you don't need to attain perfect inner harmony, or anything like it, in order to be in a good relationship. You can learn on the job. The even better news is that you don't need a relationship in order to be whole. Either way, in or out of a committed relationship, we can utilise our current situation to water our internal Garden of Eden.

This chapter specifically focuses on some fundamental Tantric meditations and exercises to nurture your own inner wholeness, aliveness and joy. They are all solo practices, equally relevant to individuals in committed relationships and single people, who wish to nurture their own sense of wholeness.

YOUR INNER LOVER

We all know that we 'should' love ourselves. But what exactly is self-love, and how do we do it? This is a huge question, and I shall be addressing different aspects of it throughout the book. I like to think of it as the ongoing process of peeling back the layers of patterning from the past that obscure our self-esteem and deepest truth. But we don't have to go excavating. When we clearly decide that we are ready to allow more love into ourselves, what will inevitably pop up are the resistances living within us that have a different agenda. As they emerge from hiding into the light of our awareness and play themselves out in our lives, we have a chance to see more clearly what they are and where they came from. Then we can choose whether to continue in our old ways or to start afresh.

One excellent way to 'grow' our love is to remember it. In shamanic traditions, where the emphasis is on reclaiming and developing personal power, it is often said that our greatest adversary is forgetfulness; forgetting our deeper truth, potential and love. However miserable our childhoods or adult lives have been, we have all, at some time, been touched by love.

Inner love meditation

The inner love meditation helps you to remember the love and beauty that you have tasted, the love and beauty inside of you.

The Technique

You'll need about twenty minutes when you will be undisturbed. Some very soft background music without words is an option, if it helps you to disengage from the outside world and to relax into yourself. Find a comfortable position either sitting or lying down. If you suspect that you could become so relaxed as to fall asleep, sit up.

- Begin with a namaste. You can either greet yourself in a mirror with your eyes open, or else close your eyes while doing the gesture, holding the intention of acknowledging Divine Love in you.

- With your eyes closed, take some relaxed, full, deep breaths, exhaling with a sigh.

- As you continue to breathe, imagine that you are breathing in and out through your heart. Place your hands over your heart energy centre (in the centre of your chest), and feel the rising and falling of your breath beneath your hands. Notice also the sensation of the warmth of your hands on your heart.

- Let your breath, arms and mind relax into a gentle awareness of love.

- Let your mind gently wander as you recall times in the past when you've felt loving, loved, at peace, at one, from childhood up to the present day. Perhaps it was a magical moment alone in the silent expanse of nature. Maybe you recall special times with a parent or grandparent or special friend. As an adult, you may remember an exquisite sexual experience alone or with a partner, or a tender and intimate time with your beloved.

- You can allow one memory to lead on to another, until your attention comes to rest on one particular event.

- Immerse yourself in recalling that occasion. What were you doing? Was anyone with you? What was happening around you? What were you seeing, hearing, smelling, tasting, touching? What feelings were evoked in you? Recall in your body the feelings and sensations of that time.

- Breathe into those feelings and sensations, sensing them in you here and now, as you rest in the warm bath of love.

- Don't worry if you feel that you are only partially able to re-enter the experience. Welcome even the smallest hints of warm or expansive feelings. There's no need to go looking for anything else or trying to do anything different. Just relax and appreciate what is actually here now.

- If the memory that comes to mind involves, for example, a partner with whom you have subsequently experienced pain and grief, you can allow the feelings of sadness, anger or fear that thinking about this person evokes to come to you. Allowing yourself to really feel the pain of love lost can allow the love that is beneath it to emerge once more. However, don't dwell or ruminate on negative events. Once you have felt the painful feelings fully, bring your mind gently back to the beautiful moments.

- As you soak up and saturate your body and mind with love, touch a part of your body that feels warm, alive, relaxed or spacious, in other words anywhere that you feel a sense of well-being, as you do this.

- Consciously let this gesture of touching yourself in this place and in this way become a way into, an anchor back to that past experience of love. Now, and at any time in the future when you want a 'shot of love', you can return to this memory and the feelings that it re-evokes in you, by repeating the gesture.

- As you practise returning to this inner place of love, you will strengthen and deepen your ability to be 'in love' at will. Naturally, some days you'll feel more readily able to celebrate the joys of life, whereas on other occasions, in the midst of grief or despair, nothing could be further from your awareness. Nonetheless, like water passing over rock, every time you recall the flow of love, be it a stream or a torrent, its waters will caress the cold, hard and unfeeling places in you. Eventually love's groove will be impossible to erase.

- When you are ready, finish with a namaste and open your eyes.

LIBERATING SEXUAL ENERGY

In the English language, we sometimes equate the word 'sexual' with 'genital', which assumes that sex happens only in the genitals. This need not be the case. 'Better sex' does not necessarily entail more intense genital experiences; deep fulfilment happens when love and sexual pleasure unite, infusing the whole of the body and being.

Tantra is often seen as a series of techniques that can be mastered in order to have better, longer-lasting and more spiritual sex. Whereas practising Tantra can and does result in all of these benefits, they are natural by-products of choosing Tantra as an attitude and a way of life, more than the consequence of 'doing' a certain technique. In fact, many of the 'techniques' in Tantra consist of a process of undoing all the work we've done, mostly on an unconscious level, to inhibit and control our natural life-force energy.

Some of us were not adequately nurtured as babies. Perhaps as children we were 'too much' for our parents in our constant curiosity and excitement about life, in our unrestrained emotional responses to pleasure and pain. As adolescents and young adults we may have fallen in love, given ourselves totally, and then been harshly disillusioned or betrayed. For whatever reason, at some time or other, we either consciously or unconsciously decided that we would never experience that degree of pain again. In accordance with that decision, we developed strategies for disconnecting our minds from our bodies at times of stress, or tightening up our musculature to protect the vulnerable softness underneath. Whereas, in our development, these defence mechanisms were a necessary strategy for insulating us from further insults and injuries, sadly they also reduced our capacity to feel the heights of pleasure, joy and bliss. Many of us continue in this way well into adulthood. We succeed in becoming, as the Pink Floyd song goes, 'comfortably numb'.

If we want to feel more in sex and in love, then we need to unbuckle our suits of armour, call our spirit back home to the body, and be open to feeling more across the board – more anger, more grief, more fear, more love, more joy, more bliss, more ecstasy. That's the deal.

'If you can't be ecstatic in anger, then you can't be ecstatic in love,' says Margot Anand, one of my teachers. The word 'ecstasy' means to 'stand outside' our small selves, and by default experience a wider perspective on life. When we're ecstatic we're fully in life, not judging or qualifying our experiences as good or bad. We're fully here, just being alive.

Kundalini shaking

Kundalini shaking helps us to let go of our unseen shackles of rigidity in body, feelings and mind, and offers us a new lease of life. Kundalini literally means 'coiled serpent', and it is the word used by Eastern mystics to describe the full potential of our sexual life-force energy to infuse the whole of our being. Kundalini shaking opens up the constrictions of bodily tension and frozen emotions, through, as its name suggests, shaking, to make way for a clear flow of energy throughout the body. Once the container of the body has been prepared and is available to receive energy flow, it will come. We do not need to go looking for it. When we allow a free-flow of energy inside ourselves, we are able to feel more, be more of who we really are and experience greater love and connection with others and deeper peace.

Kundalini shaking is a wonderful way to settle back into yourself when you return home from work, and a great way to wake yourself up and feel more alive and invigorated at the start of a Tantric date.

> ### *The Technique*
>
> You'll need about ten to twenty minutes, and if you're a woman a supportive bra may increase your comfort during this exercise. Some appropriately 'shaky' music is helpful (*see* Resources, *page 250*, for suggestions).
>
> - Put on the music.
>
> - Stand upright, barefoot if possible, with your feet about shoulder-width apart, soles flat on the ground and knees bent.
>
> - Close your eyes and take some deep breaths into your belly, exhaling with a sigh. Breathe through your mouth, and let your jaw be relaxed. How we hold our jaw is generally a reflection of how we hold the muscles and energy in our pelvis. So,

whenever you remember, let go of any tension in your jaw and in your pelvic floor, to facilitate a whole-body energy flow. (*See page 116* for further information on the pelvic floor muscles and sexual energy.)

- Imagine that you're standing on a vibrating platform, and that this vibrating platform is causing your knees to shake. Moving both knees together, allow a gentle, relaxed, rapid bouncing motion to arise in your legs, both legs moving together. This motion is entirely different from the controlled motion of an exercise class. Another image that might be helpful is to imagine you're in a bus driving on a cobbled street. It's that fast, trembling kind of experience.

- Let the shaking in your knees spread to your hips and pelvis. Let your pelvis shake and vibrate. Don't worry about how you look – that's unimportant, and there's no one looking anyway! The main point is how you feel. Look for a sense of freedom, of spontaneity.

- Notice any time when you're holding yourself back, either in your body (you may be squeezing your buttocks, for example, and limiting your range of pelvic movement), or in your mind (you might be thinking 'I can't do that!' and 'I'd look ridiculous' or 'I'm totally uncoordinated, so what's the use anyway?' or 'What would the neighbours/my friends/my mother think?'). Experiment with letting go just that little bit more.

- Let the shaking extend up to your torso and spine. Relax your spine and find the natural undulation initiated by the vibration in your knees.

- Shake out your arms and hands. Include your shoulders, loosening up any tension that you feel here.

- Surrender your head to the motion of your body. Imagine it's a duck bobbing up and down on the waves of your body's motion.

- Remember to soften your jaw and your pelvic floor (did they tighten up while all the rest of your body was letting go?), and let your whole body be fluid and floppy like a rag doll, as you 'shake it all out'.

- As you shake your physical body, imagine that you're shaking off anything that's holding you back in your life. Release stress and anger, limiting beliefs and ingrained patterns. Wave goodbye to work, office politics, problems to solve, things to be done.

- Give a sound to whatever you're feeling. If you're frustrated, growl or shout, letting the sound emerge from deep within you (rather than forcing a noise from your throat). If you're sad or upset, whimper or cry. If you're embarrassed, make a shy or nervous sound. If you feel liberated and joyful, sing, hoot or laugh. You may not be feeling anything in particular, in which case just let any sound come out, loosening up your throat and expressing your glorious free spirit.

- After about seven to ten minutes of active shaking, start experimenting with letting go of as much effort as possible while remaining upright and continuing to vibrate. Soften your body even more than before, becoming more receptive, and let the shaking shake you. Explore that place where it feels as though you are being moved, shaken, vibrated, undulated, and you're not having to do anything.

- The motion may be more subtle and internal, or larger and more visceral. The amplitude of physical motion may vary in a wave-like manner. Just follow wherever the vibration takes you. This is your life-force energy, your aliveness, your orgasmic energy flowing through you.

- If there's anywhere in your body that still feels tight, tense, painful, hard or numb, place one or both hands lightly on that part, sending it love and acceptance. Do not try to make it go away; simply notice where you are stiffening up, and if you're able, practise letting go bit by bit.

- Then return your attention to a part of your body that feels open, free, alive and in motion. Celebrate that you have a body that can move and feel, that can bring you pleasure in life.

- Gradually allow your outer movement to become smaller and finer, staying soft, relaxed and receptive.

- Notice what is still moving on the inside, perhaps a vibration, a warmth or buzzing, a sense of lightness and expansiveness, or any other sensations or feelings.

- In your own time, keeping 60 per cent of your attention on your bodily sensations, open your eyes.

- This is the completion of kundalini shaking. You can either end here with a namaste, or move on to another meditation or lovemaking with your partner.

When you have practised kundalini shaking a few times, you may also like to explore the full, one-hour-long kundalini meditation, available on CD (*see* Resources, *page 250*). This involves three further stages: dancing, sitting listening to music, and sitting or lying down in silence.

Some people naturally and immediately fall in love with kundalini shaking and find that they want to shake lots more.

> *At my first Diamond Light Tantra workshop, doing the kundalini shaking was like finding an old friend. I was able to let go, and 'let the shaking shake me'. And then it could carry on, infusing the whole of my body with pleasurable vibrations. It can be difficult to let go of control, and accept the challenges of facing my fear of losing control, and my guilt about really being an alive sexual being just for myself. In doing so, the healing for me has been a greater willingness to accept myself and to be myself: not to be the person others think I should be or even who I think I should be. To be the true person that I am.*
>
> RICHARD, 40, IT CONSULTANT

For others, their first experience of kundalini shaking can be a bit more mysterious, as the account below shows.

> *When the exercise was first demonstrated, I thought, 'I can't do that!' It looked so uninhibited (and I was a bit embarrassed), and I couldn't work out how you got from shaking to the involuntary vibrations ('let the shaking shake you', I was told). Anyway, I gave it a go, without a lot of expectation. After a while, though, I could feel subtle ripples moving through me, like little wavelets of warmth, though it wasn't exactly warm. It felt nice, like being in a bubbling stream. My back became quite sore, where I'd had problems for years. Strangely, it got worse and worse and worse, and then the pain went! What remained stiff as a brick was my neck. Apparently that's quite common for 'heady' people, and that's me. That's why I'm doing Tantra, to get out of my head.*
>
> GERRY, 52, FINANCIAL ADVISER

You can think of your body as a vessel for the transportation of energy, like a hosepipe that hasn't been used for a long time. As it's languished idle in the garden, dirt, dust, soil and moss have found their way inside.

Little creatures have made their homes in its dry interior, and have imported still more debris. Then, all of a sudden, you turn on the tap. Initially, there are going to be some impediments to the flow of water, as it judders and splutters, dislodging the protesting insect inhabitants and their homes. After a while, though, the flow becomes smoother and more uniform. This is what it can be like practising kundalini shaking. So whether you're effortlessly and blissfully vibrating in harmony with the universe, or whether your shoulders are aching terribly, you're perfectly on course!

Two fundamental principles involved in the practice of Diamond Light Tantra are worth mentioning here. These are *allowing* and *grounding*. The more that we are fully willing to allow ourselves to be touched by life, by sexual, relational and energetic experiences, without losing touch with ourselves, our truth and integrity, our authority and self-worth, which are our ground, then the greater capacity we have to open up to more of who we really are.

In the above quotes, where a pleasurable experience of kundalini shaking happened, the practitioners were relaxing and softening their bodies in order to be fully available to the energetic movements inside them. They were neither pushing to reach a particular goal or outcome, nor tensing up in resistance to what was happening inside themselves. This is what I mean by 'allowing'. Allowing has mental and emotional components as well as physical ones. A mental attitude of allowing means being prepared to let go of predetermined ideas of what a particular event should look or feel like. Emotional allowing entails a willingness to feel whatever feeling presents itself, again without judgement.

Being grounded is about having your roots deeply embedded in the earth, of having firm foundations from which to build your tower to the skies. Although heaven on earth sounds pretty appealing to most of us, the mundane and the terrible aspects of being embodied in human form are less attractive. For this reason, many of us choose to inhabit our bodies, or at least the lower parts of them, only as much as we have to. The disadvantage of being, in this way, less 'grounded' is that we miss the good bits too, and feel somehow disconnected from the rest of humanity, our home, country and the marvels of nature. We may also find it difficult to hold our own in the face of strong influences. Being grounded requires a capacity to feel; it offers strength, stability and resourcefulness. Here you have the basis for a deeply, increasingly fulfilling life.

CHAPTER FIVE

(INTIMATE RELATIONSHIP AS A SPIRITUAL PATH)

Tantra is a path of contact. Through intimate contact we can see ourselves more clearly. It was in relationship (or through lack of adequate early relationships) that many of our difficulties with intimacy arose, and it is in relationship that they can be healed – if we know how, and are willing to look clearly at the reflection of ourselves that relationships offer us.

We think that we will find wholeness if we find the right partner. In fact, it is the other way around: we find the right partner who, by failing to make us whole, shows us where we still need to find wholeness in ourselves. 'Looking in the mirror' entails redirecting the finger that you are pointing at your partner, the finger that says 'you ... ', and instead pointing the finger back at yourself and saying 'I ... '. Relationships offer us plenty of opportunities to see parts of ourselves that we tend to keep hidden, even from ourselves – both those aspects that we fear, dislike or judge, and also our beauty, light and brilliance. By reintegrating these qualities, we become more complete.

Before we met, when Roger was praying for an intimate relationship, he sent this message to the Universe: 'God, please bring me a relationship that isn't boring.' Then I showed up. Having been a serious and subdued provincial doctor for much of his adult life, Roger tracked down a hot-blooded north London Jewish princess with a sharp tongue and lightning-quick temper. I was to be his mirror. My job was to show him his passion, simply by being me.

To begin with, Roger loved my passionate nature, which awoke and inspired his. He adored my lustful advances and my forthright way of declaring my own perspective as unequivocal fact. After a while, however, he became less enthusiastic. I shouted, screamed and cried at him whenever he was distant, too cool or in any other way unavailable. He hated it. He had fallen in love with a playful, spontaneous, light-hearted sensual woman, and before his eyes I had transmogrified into a raging banshee. His response to this assault on his senses was to withdraw still further, to rise above it all, to become as cool as clear mountain air, to go away and meditate, to pretend it didn't matter, that he hadn't heard me, that he had something else important to do.

Of course, there's nothing a banshee hates more than a man who disregards her screeching. When we met and our eyes had locked in a profound, timeless gaze, I knew that finally here was a man with deep, unflinching presence – a man who would travel with me to the ends of the earth and who would not abandon me. Yet here he was, only two years later, ascending in a whiff of divine luminosity to a land where my words could no longer reach him. I felt lonely and powerless, hurt and disappointed.

At this point in a relationship, it's very tempting to call it a day. When your beloved soulmate becomes your very own rat from hell, the last thing you want is some idealistic idiot telling you that this relationship is your spiritual path. It can take an almighty leap of faith, the knowledge of how much you have invested in being with your partner, or the still-echoing memories of true love, to embrace the possibility that your partner could be offering you a great gift by being exactly as they are. It's not easy, but that quantum shift in perspective can transform your whole reality.

BEYOND DUALITY

As discussed previously (*see page 22*), the Tantric greeting of namaste is a gesture that can remind us to recognise another person, in this case your partner, as a reflection of yourself. It is an invitation to move beyond duality. We are used to seeing pleasure and pain as originating 'out there'. In relationships, we can be quick to blame our partner for our disappointments, expecting them to provide us with the gifts they showed us when we first met, which is why we bought them in the first place. Oops – got together with them. The real gift, in the disappointment, is to recognise that the pain that we imagine to be caused by our partner is actually inside us already. This means that the pleasure and joy are also in us, and we can bring them back. Now there is hope.

Receptive gaze

Receptive gaze is a way of looking inwards, through receiving the impressions, feelings, and experiences that arise in us when we let the outside world touch us. It is about receiving through the windows of our eyes. It is also a way of allowing our true selves to be seen by another. Receptive gaze allows us, when shared with another, to feel our own feelings more deeply, and to own them as ours. In this way we are able to notice the feelings that obscure our flow of love, and to allow ourselves to melt down into our loving essence. In this way we can appreciate the world, and our beloved, more fully.

I'm sure you've already heard that the eyes are windows of the soul. Unfortunately, though, for many of us, these windows are in desperate need of cleaning. Clouded by the dust of time and unconsciousness, we can allow certain aspects of ourselves (usually those that we imagine will be socially acceptable) to be seen, and we see outside ourselves, but not the whole picture. We have forgotten, are frightened to be real, be true, be open, be love. This, in the words of Kahlil Gibran, is '... the seasonless world where you shall laugh, but not all of your laughter, and weep, but not all of your tears'.

Receptive gazing is a form of inner window cleaning that enables our eyes to openly reflect our true selves. It is not goal orientated; it is an exploration, a meditation. In receptive gazing, your awareness is primarily located inside your own body, in contact with the sensations and feelings within. Your eyes are in soft focus, not looking at or for anything in particular. You breathe and welcome your responses to what you see, and allow yourself to feel and to receive the fullness of sight and experience. You allow yourself to be seen.

Receptive gaze alone can be particularly enjoyable when you are outdoors in nature. The separation between you and the environment can gradually soften, and you may be able to more fully appreciate the beauty and wonder in nature and your essential connectedness as a living being.

The Technique

You can enter into receptive gazing whenever, and for as long as you choose. Allow yourself from two to twenty minutes.

- Close your eyes, take some deep breaths and exhale with a sound or sigh.

- As you breathe, bring your attention back to your body. Notice any tension in your body, and as you breathe, gently allow any part of you that is willing to do so to let go.

- Become aware of any sensations or feelings in your body. Notice your breath coming in and going out.

- Open your eyes, slowly and gently, letting 80 per cent of your attention remain with your body sensations and feelings, as you continue to breathe.

Intimate relationship as a spiritual path

- Being present in your body is an anchor to being here and now, not in your mind, which is busy thinking about either the past or the future. You may also like to become aware of the place between your eyebrows in your forehead known as the third eye, the eye that looks inwards.

- Gently receive the sights that enter your eyes, letting your eyeballs stay relaxed and natural, without staring or straining.

- Notice any bodily sensations or feelings that arise as you do this. Welcome these.

Eye gazing

When we receive the eyes of another person with receptive gaze, this is called eye gazing, or soul gazing. It is an opportunity to be truly intimate with another, letting down the façades of personality and allowing ourselves to be seen as we really are.

During eye gazing you may experience a range of feelings, from boredom to frustration to sexual arousal to love and tenderness. There is no right or wrong way to feel. Keep welcoming whatever comes up, and let it be there fully. Remember the phrase 'what we resist persists', so if you are repeatedly feeling bored or irritable, ask yourself if there is something that you are trying not to feel. Also, let your feelings be simply feelings. As we take responsibility for how we are feeling, knowing that its intensity is related to previous unresolved pain, we are 'in awareness'. We can then more easily accept how we are feeling, without pushing or pulling or needing to change anything. When we really accept ourselves as we are, we are being compassionate towards ourselves. We may still be enmeshed in an emotional state, but we are also, through self-awareness, self-acceptance and self-love, cultivating a way of being that loosens the grip of old emotional patterns. This is meditation.

The Technique

Decide how long you will eye gaze for. Anything from two to twenty minutes is possible. Have some tissues nearby so that if tears come to your eyes or your nose runs, you can easily reach for a tissue without disrupting the meditation. You may like to set a soft and pleasant timer (for example, an alarm clock or mobile phone that plays you a tune), or simply estimate the time. If you like, you can put on some gentle music in the background.

- Sit comfortably opposite each other and begin with a namaste.

- With receptive gaze, allow yourself to receive each other's eyes.

- Let your eyes blink naturally whenever they need to. Breathe fully and naturally, letting go of any tension you find in your body.

- Welcome any feelings or sensations that arise. Enter into these feelings or sensations fully.

- Continue to breathe deeply and naturally, remaining in receptive gaze and aware of your body sensations and feelings.

- Notice if you are following a train of thought that is taking you away from the here and now. Come gently back to the meditation.

- You may find that you go through different layers of experience. As you welcome whatever comes, returning to receptive gaze, these will pass and eventually give way to love (though probably not on every occasion of eye gazing!).

- Finish with a namaste, and take some time to share your experiences.

Pete and I were gazing into each other's eyes, and I could see that he was struggling to keep awake. Immediately that provoked my familiar deep wound, 'He's not really interested in me. He doesn't care. I'm not really lovable.' That's how I felt during most of my childhood. I was caught up in anger and hurt, and thoughts to that effect. Afterwards, through talking, I came to see that his sleepiness may have had nothing to do with me. It's incredibly intimate to be together in this way, and I think that Pete was encountering his own 'stuff', his own painful self-beliefs and emotions from his history, but didn't know how to face it and so dozed off instead. It's like a reflex in me, taking Pete's responses personally, and reacting to them. Then I'm lost in my past, and not really here and now any more.

Jane, 50, Nurse

INTIMATE COMMUNICATION

When you meet your friend ... let the spirit in you move your lips and direct your tongue.

Kahlil Gibran, The Prophet

How can we move from recognising the parts of ourselves that we aren't so proud of, to becoming kings and queens, whole unto ourselves and ready for union? It may at first appear to be a pretty tall order. The process is a gradual one, and each time we make a choice in favour of truth and love, we become more integrated. Below are some practical suggestions for navigating this territory.

Deep listening

An invaluable tool in any relationship is deep listening. If we can genuinely hear our partner's truth while simultaneously honouring our own, then a creative synthesis of the two can occur. A key phrase to remember, if you notice that you are beginning to judge your partner, and are finding it difficult to hear what they have to say, is 'Your partner is always right'. This does not mean that you are wrong; on the contrary, you are right too. You can both be right together, even if your realities appear to be contradictory. When you move away from the belief that 'There's only enough room for one truth around here!' you widen your horizons and allow the warm breeze of compassion to once again flow between you.

The following exercise is best integrated as an ongoing part of your relationship. This will facilitate deeper intimacy and empathy in general, and will mean that you are firmly grounded in the skill of deep listening even when you have emotive topics to discuss. The exercise may appear to be rather slow and laborious, but the rewards can be immense. Many arguments and hours spent fighting can sometimes be avoided by clear, open and honest dialogue and understanding.

The Technique

Deep listening is described below. You can allocate anything from twenty minutes to an hour for the process.

- Begin with a namaste.

- Decide upon a topic on which you would like to share your feelings, needs and requests.

- Take turns in speaking, talking in 'bite size' chunks of information. Focus on your own feelings, needs and requests in relation to the topic, and preferably in connection with a specific incident. Instead of 'Whenever we go to visit your sister, *you* . . . give her far more attention and love than you give me,' choose 'Yesterday, when we were visiting your sister and she was talking about her difficulties in relation to her work, you were listening very attentively *I* . . . felt envious because I need attention too. I would love you to be that interested in my struggles at the office.'

- After you have spoken, your partner reflects back to you the essence of what they have heard you say. If they have not quite understood, repeat the phrase or segment until you are clear that they understand the bottom line of your meaning.

- Then it is your partner's turn to speak. When they have finished, you similarly repeat back the essence of what you have heard. Your partner clarifies what they have said until they are satisfied that you have heard them accurately.

- Continue in this way.

- End with a namaste.

Needs

If we are unused to recognising or accepting the truth of our actual wants, needs and desires, we may need to devote time and energy to uncovering them.

Chuck Spezzano, a renowned teacher and author in the area of personal development and relationships, says this about needs: 'We all have needs until we realise ourselves as whole and spirit ... By accepting your needs, they are naturally let go of and, as a result, a new bonding occurs. Bonding means love and success with ease ... '

Needs are part of the human condition. When we allow ourselves to be human, we paradoxically take a step closer to our essence, our divinity. When we accept and share our needs with our partner, without demanding that they fulfil them, we are being honest, open and intimate.

Appreciations

Another simple and yet invaluable tool to remember in communicating with your beloved is to appreciate them. Appreciations open our hearts and help us to recognise the beauty in our partner, and the needs, longings and desires that they do, in fact, fulfil in us. Appreciations remind us that even if the proverbial glass appears to be three-quarters empty, it is nonetheless a quarter full. Appreciations help us to focus and direct our energy towards what we want and value.

- Each day, notice two things that you have appreciated and valued in your partner that day.

- Even if you think that they know about it, tell them anyway. Nothing is too small to mention. Even everyday occurrences such as your partner taking out the rubbish or cooking dinner would become a big deal if your partner stopped doing them! Remember that it is never boring to be appreciated!

- Let them know what feelings their actions evoked in you, and which of your needs, longings or desires were fulfilled.

- Receive appreciations gracefully. Notice if you have a tendency to brush them away, or alternatively if you are willing to be touched by them. If possible, respond with 'thank you'.

AVOIDING INTIMACY: THE DISTANCER-PURSUER DANCE

We yearn for intimacy, and yet we go to great lengths to avoid it. One way to prevent intimacy, while appearing to search for it avidly, is by engaging in the distancer-pursuer dance.

This intriguing dance can continue for a lifetime. Most of us (enlightened masters aside) do it. Many of us aren't aware that we're treading in such well-worn grooves, or that there is another way. The distancer-pursuer dance may be very dramatic, heroic, tragic and engaging, but in general it's not much fun. It can be excruciatingly painful.

The distancer-pursuer dance, as its name suggests, is a pattern in which one partner chases the other, wanting more contact, communication, love or sex from them. The other partner correspondingly moves away from contact, communication, love or sex, either physically or metaphorically. At any one time, who takes which position may be pretty fixed. However, it is not uncommon for a complete reversal of roles to occur for both partners, either spontaneously or over time.

> *When we first got together six years ago, sex was amazing. I loved Helen's sauciness, and we explored lots of things and made love all the time. About a year later, I still wanted it to carry on that way, but Helen was becoming less interested in sex. She was spending a lot of time and energy in trying to lose weight and getting her career going. I was hurt by her frequent rejections, and after a while I took up sailing to get out of the house and escape from my disappointment. Now that Helen's career is pretty successful and she's slim and healthy, she's always getting at me for being so preoccupied with things and wanting me to be more intimate with her. Somehow, though, I'm just not interested any more. I just can't seem to get myself going, and when I do it's never right for her.*
>
> JOHN, 32, GRAPHIC DESIGNER

As Helen and John's story shows, there's no better place to play the game than in the bedroom. Someone on my Deep Diving Tantra training, who came to the course because he wanted sex and his wife didn't, having heard the stories of the other couples in the group, did a little home survey. 'It's incredible!' he told me over the phone. 'Of all of our close friends, almost none of the couples has compatible sex drives. Either it's the man who wants sex and the woman doesn't, or it's the other way round. It's hardly ever equal.' The mysterious world of sexual relationships clearly defies mathematical reasoning!

So why, if it's so painful and unrewarding, do we dance this dance? Painful as it is, the distancer-pursuer dance protects us from something even more frightening: the possibility of taking a step into the unknown and perhaps facing disappointment or even allowing in love.

In our own distancer-pursuer dance, I initially played the part of the pursuer. In keeping with my pattern of attraction to unavailable men, I'd chosen one who had been divorced twice and was still in the process of separating from his third long-term partner. Marriage for him represented the painfully shattered illusion of his youthful dreams.

So it was with utter frustration, and yet complete safety, that I fantasised about marriage, wrote poetry and finally proposed to this man. Roger was touched by my invitation, said that he loved me, but no – and then, after a few more drinks, yes. Deliriously happy, we went out to celebrate.

The next morning Roger was so ill that he could not get out of bed, and it wasn't just a hangover. By the time he had recovered from a severe bout of gastric flu three weeks later, he remembered nothing about my proposal, his acceptance or our night of celebration.

I was devastated. There ensued weeks, months and years of me chasing and chastising him, feeling heartbroken and wronged but clearly on the moral high ground and undoubtedly the more spiritually evolved of the two of us. Then the tables turned. He proposed to me.

At that point I really started to wobble. I remembered how absolutely Roger did not conform with my fantasy of marrying a millionaire, or at least someone moderately rich, with whom I could lead a life of luxury as a kept woman. All the times that he had let me down or disappointed me ran through my mind and jangled my emotions as if I'd been watching a several-year-long TV drama. Our age difference and his prospects for long-term health and longevity looked grim and, quite frankly, I couldn't imagine why I had ever wanted to be with him in the first place.

Basically, I was terrified of re-enacting and re-experiencing my childhood, during which I had felt anxious, overburdened with responsibility, hurt and abandoned. I was afraid of real commitment and real intimacy, because I feared that if I really opened up and trusted, I would be hurt again in the same way and to the same extent as I was as a child. In my fear, a part of me would rather suffer the known frustrations of 'a safe distance for intimacy' than risk stepping into the unknown, where I might either meet my deeper pain, or discover the possibility of deep fulfilment.

In case you are wondering, I did eventually say 'yes', still wobbling, but having connected with the longings of my heart, and valuing these above the cautions of my mind. In fact, so far, it's been a mixture of both my hopes and fears; the joy, fulfilment and pain. A journey of empowerment resulting in a blossoming of love, and sometimes ecstasy. I am truly grateful that I chose the way of my heart. Commitment provides a safe container in which our deepest fears and wounds can come to the surface for airing and transformation, and then we become freer, and more able to truly love.

In short, our fear of the unknown is often greater than our dislike of the known, imperfect status quo. In more poetic terms:

> *Our greatest fear is not that we are inadequate*
> *Our deepest fear is that we are powerful beyond measure.*
>
> MARIANNE WILLIAMSON, SPOKEN BY NELSON MANDELA IN HIS
> INAUGURATION SPEECH

Below are some tips for recognising your steps in this dance – your fears, motivations and options for finding new moves.

- Firstly, begin to observe, in your relationship, whether you habitually take the role of distancer or pursuer. You may even take on both roles in different aspects of life – for instance, you can seek more verbal communication (pursuer) and avoid sex (distancer).

- In situations where you experience yourself as the pursuer, notice and write down how you feel if you desist from chasing after your partner, while keeping your heart open to yourself and them. What are your fears, hopes, needs, desires and longings in relation to them?

- Where you find yourself in the role of distancer, similarly notice and write down how you feel if you stop moving away from your partner. Let your heart stay open to yourself and your partner, welcoming the feelings that come up. What are your fears, hopes, needs, desires and longings in the relationship?
- At a mutually agreeable moment, share these feelings with your partner.

THE DANCE OF FREEDOM AND TOGETHERNESS

We all have needs for closeness, and a need for freedom, for time alone and time apart. Often in relationships partners polarise, meaning that one person represents the need for freedom, while the other partner embodies the need for togetherness. It is a creative, dynamic tension that every individual and relationship must negotiate. By stepping out of the distancer-pursuer dance, and with intimate communication, couples can find a way to each acknowledge their own hopes and fears, needs and wants, both for freedom and for togetherness.

Tantra, in its truest expression as a path to enlightenment, is ultimately about union. It is about inner harmony and unification of all aspects of ourselves, and it is about the universal union of masculine and feminine, man and woman, Shiva and Shakti, that transcends duality. This, however, is an entirely different phenomenon from the undifferentiated merging of two people in symbiotic coexistence. It is common to confuse the two.

Tantra is unlikely to transport you back to the heady bliss that you may have felt when you first met your beloved, when you believed that through them you were at last whole, healed and happy. Tantra can, and does, support couples in finding great joy, love, bliss and ecstasy together *with* each other, not *because of* each other. For many couples this journey needs to start with each partner becoming more of a separate, individuated person in their own right.

Brian and Sarah became interested in Tantra after eight years of marriage. Initially, their relationship had been very passionate – in fact it was the first time in her life that Sarah had felt so in touch with her sexuality. Their loving passion bore fruit, and within four years they had three children.

It started gradually and imperceptibly, and yet, by their fifth anniversary, Sarah had almost entirely lost interest in sex. She sometimes did concede to Brian's sexual advances, to keep the peace and because she thought that as a wife, she 'should', but neither of them felt truly fulfilled. Brian was becoming more and more sexually frustrated, and could hardly sleep at night. Having read an article in a magazine, they decided to see if Tantra could help.

After attending a women's Tantra weekend, Sarah hardly recognised herself. She had discovered parts of herself that she didn't know were there, and in particular she had discovered her ability to say 'no' to what she didn't want sexually. Feeling empowered, inspired and disorientated, she returned home to Brian.

While Brian was interested in, intrigued by and supportive of the changes he saw in Sarah, he was also dismayed at their consequences in bed. Sarah was experiencing a lot of guilt when she refused Brian's advances, but she was saying 'no' nonetheless. She oscillated uncomfortably between her new-found authority and a lifetime of pleasing her man even if she wasn't really enjoying it. Whereas previously she had felt OK about having sex to satisfy Brian, now she felt even more deflated and out of sorts afterwards. What was also uncomfortable for her was that she had not yet discovered her 'yes'. What was it that she *did* want sexually? What if she never felt sexual again?

As far as Brian was concerned, if sexuality had been a barren landscape before, it was now the Sahara Desert. In his words: 'What on earth had we done? This new place was supposed to be cosy and comforting, whereas actually it was unknown and different, like being in the dark. What if we drifted apart or couldn't find what we had hoped for? This wasn't in the manual. I wanted my money back.'

When one or both partners in a relationship begin to recognise, either consciously or unconsciously, this need, yearning or longing to know themselves, to become whole and healed unto themselves, they may be tempted to consider that this need for freedom must necessitate the end of the relationship. Whereas for some relationships this will be the case, for many others the calling to 'know thyself' is actually the heralding of the death of the old relationship as it was, and the birth of a new relationship, with the same partner, on different grounds. Again, this need not be a jointly created new ground; it can be enough that a couple stay together and commit to negotiate this new terrain together. In doing so, when a couple commit to realising their full potential, both as individuals and together in partnership, the alchemy can begin.

Despite some initial misgivings, Brian and Sarah signed up for more workshops, this time together. Brian imagined that only Sarah would benefit, and through her, their sexual relationship could be given a new lease of life. It wasn't long, however, before he was also discovering things about himself. Of their relationship he wrote: 'Wait a minute, this place is actually getting better by the day. I'm clearer about me, and I'm clearer about you. How cool! I'm happy being me. Phew!' A little later he wrote: 'Well, fancy that – having respect and desire, love and lust together. Happier with me, more content with us. Who would have thought that we would be able to offer more, give more, and receive more; resent less, worry less and fear less?'

It had taken Sarah a long time to truly become at home with 'no', and yet once she did, she subsequently found it so easy to say 'yes'! She felt immensely appreciative of Brian's acceptance, and his welcoming of the 'new her' and willingness to weather difficulties for the sake of their relationship. Both of them were really enjoying this second honeymoon and were discovering their genuine, mutual pleasure in sexual relating.

Brian is helping Sarah by checking with her when she says 'yes' to make sure that she really means it. Sometimes it's still difficult. Says Sarah: 'Since I have found my no and now my yes I have really started to feel more and experience more and feel so connected with the rest of my body, particularly my yoni, which I have realised I have ignored and abused as much as anybody else.'

For other couples, the process of integration and harmonisation of the needs for separateness and closeness begins when one of them has, or considers having, an affair. If an affair happens, there will be much pain and loss of trust to be bridged. Ultimately, if a couple are strong enough to find a way through these choppy waters, the attraction in the affair, and any future attractions to other people, can be integrated into the relationship by means of loving communication. When we look at the qualities that we find attractive in others, we can see more clearly that these are aspects of ourselves, and of relationship, that we are longing for. This can open up a new arena of dialogue within the relationship between love partners, and can allow the relationship to reach its next stage in evolution, through including these previously missing components.

As will be clear by now, an intimate relationship need never be boring! The process of self-discovery and the unfolding of love and truth never end, as we become clearer about our own healing journey, as we see our partner for who they really are, and as we embrace our needs and longings and are able to communicate them. The more familiar we become with these tools, the easier and more joyful the journey of relationship becomes.

Rupert was three-quarters of the way through a year's Tantra course on his own when he fell in love with Natasha. Rupert, at thirty-seven, had a full and happy sexual history. His previous relationship had been fiery and passionate. Tantra had helped him to integrate his strong sexual drive with his softer, sensitive and deeply compassionate heart. He was more confident in himself in all aspects of life, and felt that he had become more of a mature man.

So, bursting with energy, he met the beautiful and delicate Natasha. Natasha had a history of betrayal from men, and was frightened to trust them. She saw Rupert's involvement with Tantra as a threat, and wondered what he was getting up to with other women. Although they were already living together in Rupert's studio flat, they had so far not had sexual intercourse. 'I can't believe it!' Rupert shared at a workshop, 'I'm in love with a woman who doesn't like sex!' His compassion and patience were wearing thin at the seams as his sexual frustration, despite his Tantric experience, became difficult to contain.

After much soul searching and little success in enticing Natasha into the world of Tantra, Rupert realised that he couldn't keep blaming his frustration and disappointment on Natasha, and that he would have to find a new place of resourcefulness in himself. He decided to really listen to Natasha, and to become aware of any rigid or limiting aspects of himself. As a result of this, he discovered that he had labelled Natasha as 'a woman who doesn't like sex', and that this attitude was self-perpetuating. He decided to change his outlook.

Rupert opened up to the possibility that Natasha was a woman who loved sex, and to his surprise he became frightened. He came face to face with his fear of intimacy, which had, up to that point, been kept at bay by their lack of sexual contact and his attitude of blame. Rupert decided to communicate to Natasha his fear of real intimacy, and his commitment to work through it with her. This opened up a doorway in their relationship, and pretty soon they were making love fully and integrating Tantra into their sexual relating. I remember his pride in sharing in the Tantra group what a 'damn fine girlfriend' he had!

INTIMACY

Committed relationships offer us ongoing opportunities to be truly intimate. Intimacy, or 'into-me-see', is far more that a close cuddle or an erotic embrace. Intimacy is about being real. Intimacy is about having the courage to see another human being as they are, not as a replica of our past or as who we want them to be. Intimacy entails revealing ourselves, being naked in more than just the physical sense, and making space in ourselves to welcome another as they reveal themselves. It is about making love with the lights on, in the bedroom and inside ourselves, and with our eyes open.

As we move through the protective barriers that conceal our true selves, we move closer to our essence, our true nature, our essential oneness with all beings that is love.

CHAPTER SIX

TANTRIC PRINCIPLES IN LOVEMAKING AND IN LIFE

'Tantra changed my life!'
ANNIE, 38, VIDEO PRODUCER

Tantra is a life path. How we make love is how we create the life we lead, and vice versa. This chapter outlines some of the principles of Tantra, which can be incorporated into lovemaking as well as into any other aspect of life.

A child is totally dependent on his or her caregivers for basic survival. If parenting is inadequate, or other disruptive or traumatic events occur, the only way for children to protect themselves from unmanageable discomfort is in some way to distance their awareness from, or block off, the pain. If, as adults, we have not developed more mature coping strategies, or if we encounter overwhelming life events, we continue with this process of creating 'energy blocks'. These 'energy blocks' are distributed in the cells of the body, according to the energetic principles of the 'chakras' described in the next chapter. The Tantric principles in this chapter assist the process of 'unblocking' this unavailable energy, and utilising it optimally. When our energy, our resources and our capabilities in life are flowing freely, the benefits are equally applicable in sex as in the whole of life. For each Tantric principle that I outline, I offer explanations and exercises to give you a flavour of its potential in both arenas – life as a whole and sex.

EXPANSION

Tantra is about expansion. This means accessing and embodying our fullest potential. Physical expansion corresponds with relaxation in the body, a deep breath, a sense of peace, aliveness and well-being. Emotional expansion means shedding repetitive patterns of negativity and pain, and finding hope, love, compassion and beauty. Mental expansion entails breaking out of limiting belief systems and getting creative. Spiritual expansion means opening to deeper levels of truth, love and connectedness.

In lovemaking and in life, we can learn to recognise expansion and its opposite, contraction, in ourselves. Below are some tools to support us in living from a place of greater expansion.

AWARENESS

As I have already mentioned, awareness is one of the fundamental principles in Tantra. We have the choice, at any moment, to become attentive to our thoughts, feelings, impulses and physicality, and in this way to become more aware of ourselves. Simply by becoming aware of our moment-by-moment thoughts, feelings and body sensations, we allow change to happen naturally. Our body and being wants to find balance and harmony. By shining the torch of awareness on the dark areas of our inner worlds, we gradually bring more light into our lives.

Awareness in life

Try this short exercise to demonstrate the powerful effect of attention, and through attention bodily awareness.

> ### The Technique
>
> You can do this exercise while waiting in the queue at the supermarket, or at any other moment that takes your fancy. It will take about three minutes.
>
> - Stand, sit or lie down comfortably, and close your eyes. Breathe comfortably, deeply and naturally.
>
> - As you breathe, give all your attention to your right hand. Notice any feelings or sensations that arise there.
>
> - See or sense your right hand in your mind's eye.
>
> - Carry on bringing your attention back in a relaxed and gentle way to your right hand for about two minutes.
>
> - Notice any changes or developments in the subtle sensations that you feel.
>
> - Open your eyes, and bring your awareness for a moment to both hands. Do they feel any different?

Generally speaking, by simply bringing our attention to something, this allows energy to move more freely, without us doing anything more than that. I would imagine that after two minutes, your right hand felt a bit different from the left one, perhaps more tingly or warm, lighter or heavier, or even larger than before. This is the power of awareness: by simply noticing what's here now, something changes.

This approach can also allow you to become more aware of other people, which has the capacity to enhance your relationship with them, as this account shows:

> *I was training to be a dance teacher over a period of three years with the same group of trainees. One time when we were dancing, I felt a great sense of warmth from one of my dancing friends, and I asked him, 'Tim, are you loving me more than usual, or what?' 'No,' he said, 'I love you just as much as I did.' He paused. 'But, you know what, I did decide to pay more attention to you. And as I become more aware of you, I feel more appreciative to have you as my friend.'*
>
> SUE, 47, DANCE TEACHER

Awareness in sex

Where is your attention when you are making love? Is it on your partner and their pleasure? On trying to have or delay an orgasm? Are you wondering whether your tummy is too big or whether the children might hear you? How about becoming aware of the here and now, in the form of your vajra or yoni? How might it be to become fully engaged, moment by moment, on the sensations in your sexual organs, to feel them fully?

Have a go at making love and every now and then pausing, and simply relaxing, breathing and feeling the sensations in your vajra or yoni. As you resume movement, notice what happens to the sensations in your genitals, and how you are thinking and feeling. Again pause, relax and breathe. Rest a while and feel into your vajra or yoni once more. Wherever possible remain in eye contact with your partner during lovemaking and while resting together, with vajra still inside yoni, in stillness. Eye contact helps you to also be aware of your beloved, while being rooted in your own experience of your sexual feelings. Every now and then you can also place a hand on your partner's heart area, to bring your awareness and theirs to your loving heart connection.

This is not a means to an end, so in making love in this way you are not aiming for any particular outcome. You can regard it as an experiment to see what difference it makes for you and your beloved when you make love and remain aware of your physical sensations, your love and your connection with each other in the here and now. This is the basis of truly relating with another human being, where you become as fully present as possible in each moment, rather than planning the future, sinking back into the past, or fantasising about something that isn't actually happening. Planning, ruminating, predicting and fantasising all happen in the head. They take you away from intimacy. Through entering deeply into your sensations and feelings in each moment, you may find yourself feeling at the same time peaceful and yet vibrating with aliveness, or even perhaps glimpsing ecstasy.

> *We were experimenting with making love without coming close to having an orgasm. This meant that we spent quite a bit of time just relaxing, breathing and feeling. I became much more aware of the subtle sensations and energetic movements within me, and between my partner and I. It was absolutely fascinating. It didn't feel at all like an absence, more like an opening up of something else. We felt so connected afterwards, and ready for more!*
>
> DALIA, 43, PSYCHOTHERAPIST

INTENT

Energy follows intent. By clarifying, unifying and mobilising your intent, you can facilitate the flow of energy in your body and in your life. By aligning your mind, feelings and actions with your higher purpose or true intent, you mobilise your will and effect greater transformation and wholeness. Clear, integrated intent can also be thought of as 'the will of the heart'. It is the love of and longing for freedom and truth.

> *... the moment one definitely commits oneself*
> *then providence moves too.*
>
> GOETHE

Intent in life

The subject of clarifying and unifying your intent is a huge and important one, which I just touch upon here. I invite you to consider the possibility that very often, when you're not getting something that you want in life, your intent may not be clear or unified. To take an example from my own life, there were a couple of years, subsequent to splitting up with my first Tantric partner in Australia, during which I was single. I thought that I clearly wanted to find another partner in the UK, and to forge a committed, long-term relationship with them. I felt rather sorry for myself because this did not seem to be happening. Meanwhile I had several beautiful but short-lived connections with men who were as a rule creative, spiritual, penniless, itinerant, foreign and free-spirited. Eventually it occurred to me that my associations with the archetype of 'marriage' (long-term, committed relationship) were predominantly pretty negative. I had grown up with the experience and perception that marriage was about stagnation and the subordination of each individual's will, integrity, authority, love and creative expression. In other words, I saw marriage as an inner death. It was hardly surprising, therefore, that I was emitting mixed messages. I was pretty shocked by that realisation, but it certainly helped me to clarify and unify my intent. Soon after I had done this, I met Roger, my husband.

Whenever you aren't achieving what you want in life, first ask yourself this question: 'What are my associations from the past (even if I no longer adhere to this viewpoint) with the thing that I want?' Then ask yourself: 'If I was to obtain what I desire, what new challenges would I need to face?'

Having clarified your intent, that is the will of your heart and spirit, rather than the will of your mind, you can concentrate on mobilising it, on bringing it into action. For example, if your intention is to slow down and feel more, you may wish to rearrange your life to have more free time for yourself, and to remind yourself of the benefits of slowing down and feeling more by keeping a journal or spending time and talking with like-minded people.

Intent in sex

At the beginning of your Tantric date with your beloved, after sharing a namaste together, take a moment to share your intent for your time together. Your intent is your guiding principle, your focus, your mantra during your time together. It is something that you can remember and recommit to at any time during the date. An intention is not about another person, which is more of a wish. For example, if you want your partner to open up to you more, you need to remember that in the end, only they can decide to do that. However, you can observe your typical reactions when your partner does not behave how you would like them to. Then your intent may be to do something different, such as opening up to them, sharing your pain at the lack of connection that you feel, rather than shouting at or criticising them.

Simple, easy to implement intentions for lovemaking or Tantric practice may be to breathe fully and deeply, to communicate honestly your thoughts and feelings, needs and desires as you make love, to let your partner's love touch you as deeply as possible or to stay as present in each moment as possible. Radhika has this story to tell.

> *When I began to practise Tantra, it opened all sorts of doors for me in my sexuality. In my previous marriage, it was straightforward bread-and-butter sex, or none at all. Since Tantra and meeting Patrick, my horizons widened beyond belief. I began trying out all sorts of new things to see how they felt, and how I felt with Patrick as we explored. I became a wild woman!*

After a while, though, I realised that I tended to be the one initiating sex, and that Patrick had become more passive. I realised that I was more strongly in touch with my proactive, 'masculine' sexual energy, and less connected with my 'feminine', receptive side. I decided to try something new. When making love with Patrick, I chose an intention, for a month, to simply receive him, to see what that was like. I wanted to move about as little as possible, and to allow my yoni to open like a beautiful cavern, and to sense his masculinity. I loved it! I felt as if I was the earth, welcoming the Sky God inside me.

Being still, open and receptive, I experienced gentle waves of bliss moving through me, but few genital orgasms. I didn't really miss them, although a little voice would pop into my head occasionally and say 'What about me?' Then I reminded myself that I have had plenty of orgasms in my life, but far fewer experiences of my receptive femininity. I knew I could have orgasms any time I wanted, by moving my body in the ways that I knew. Mostly, that month, I chose to return to my intention, enjoying the stillness and beauty of just being, feeling and letting Patrick in, and I would not have had the same depth of experiences if I hadn't.

RADHIKA, 45, ARTS MANAGER

BREATH

The way in which you breathe affects every aspect of your life. Your breath is the bridge between your body, feelings and thoughts, your energy, your past and your present. How we breathe directly affects every cell of our body, and it also influences how we feel emotionally. As such, the breath is also a vehicle for expansion and ecstasy. This section gives you a taste of how this works.

Breathing in life

I remember a simple exercise that I did as part of my training in working with the breath. The exercise involved a rebounder, a mini trampoline. We were asked to walk across the floor, take a step onto the rebounder, and then keep walking. Of course, stepping onto a rebounder is rather different from walking on a carpet. It sinks underneath your feet, wobbles a little and springs you up in the air. As the other students and I walked along the carpet, our breath was relaxed and even. When it came to stepping onto the rebounder, we all held our breath. When we returned to the carpet, we resumed normal breathing.

What we learned was that we had a habit of holding our breath when the going got tough. We braced ourselves for difficulty, hoping to lessen the blow. In fact, however, when we repeated the exercise, this time consciously breathing as we stepped onto and off the rebounder, our movements became easier and more fluid, and we felt more confident and stable. Breathing fully helps you to be more relaxed, present and energised. You have more resources available to you. Breathing through a difficult experience generally requires retraining to enable you to feel the fear and do it anyway, to the best of your ability, rather than effectively closing your eyes and hoping for the best.

Full body breathing

The following exercise shows you how to maximise your potential for deep breathing. As well as keeping you more balanced in stressful situations, full body breathing can help you to soften up energetic blocks, and to differentiate the physical, emotional and mental effects of different breathing styles. When your breath flows freely within you, you can choose to breathe fully and with consciousness. This allows you to maximise pleasurable experiences and to let them infuse the whole of your body.

Full body breathing is about unlearning our habits of reducing the flow of breath and life in our bodies, and letting go of our patterns of tension. Most of us chronically diminished the flow of our life-force energy early in life, when we experienced ongoing painful events and reducing our capacity to feel was a necessary survival strategy. However, when we feel less, we feel less pleasure in the same proportion as we feel less pain. Then we wonder where all the passion went.

The Technique

- Lie down on your back, so as to be completely relaxed. Place your hands on your belly, and let your belly rise and fall with your breath. Explore letting your breath expand your abdomen as you breathe in, and letting it deflate as you breathe out (see illustration 1 below).

- Place your hands on the sides of the bottom of your rib cage (halfway between your armpit and your hipbone). As you inhale, first feel your belly expanding, then feel the lateral movement of your ribcage under your hands. Simply relax on the exhalation.

- Place your hands on your upper chest. As you breathe in, first feel your belly, then your lateral ribcage, and then your upper chest, inflate and expand with your in-breath. Simply relax on the exhalation (see illustration 2).

- As you breathe in and out, notice any feelings or sensations that arise in you. As you open, relax and release the diaphragm you may become conscious of any feelings of vulnerability that you have held tightly stored away in your midriff. This is an opportunity to soften, accept and release whatever you find.

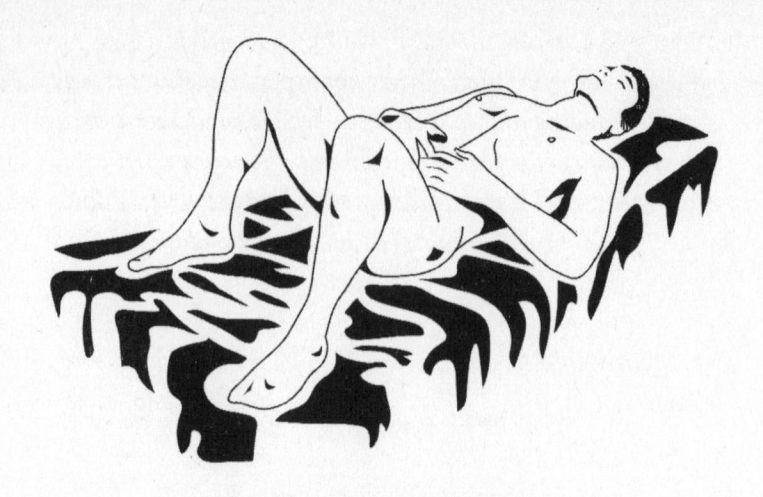

1. FULL BODY BREATHING

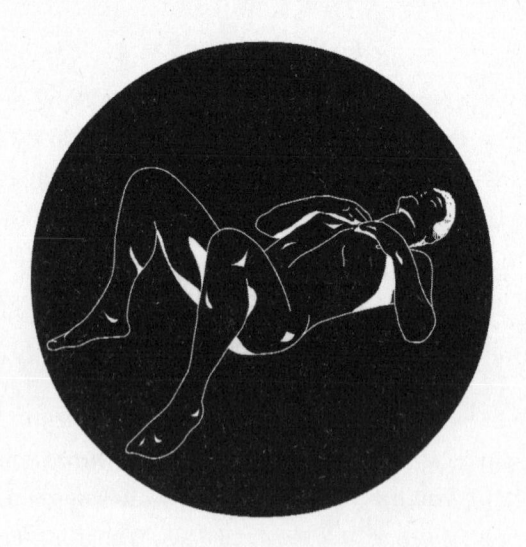

2. PLACE YOUR HANDS ON YOUR UPPER CHEST

> That first workshop had a massive impact on me. I had no real expectations, but when we were doing the 'streamings' exercise, breathing and letting vibrations of energy flow through our bodies, I felt a blockage in my chest area. I could

> *feel ripples coming up from my legs and pelvis, rising up through my belly, and then stopping at my chest. It was becoming more and more uncomfortable, and Leora came over to support me. She put her hand over my chest area, and encouraged me to breathe into it, and to relax. I don't quite know how it happened, but a tremendous wave of emotion came over me, and I started to cry for the first time in years. I can't put into words the release I felt. It was as if I had been able to put down a heavy load I'd been carrying. It was like a doorway opening, something I'd known but never before experienced.*
>
> Steven, 43, Company Director

Breathing in sex

Breathing more fully enables you to deepen your experience of pleasure and to allow pleasure to expand into love and bliss. When you hold your breath and contract the muscles in your thighs and belly, then any experience of genital arousal will be held purely in the pelvis. If, however, you breathe more fully, involving the whole of the diaphragm, with a relaxed belly and thighs, then this pleasure is able to infuse other parts of your anatomy and being.

> *My partner was stroking my body and my vajra before making love. I felt very loved, yummy and turned on. The next thing I remember is her saying, 'You've stopped breathing. What's going on for you?' I had been lost in thoughts, and her words brought me back into my body. After a few more minutes the same thing happened again, and then I decided to open my eyes in order to stay more present with her. She encouraged me to take a deep breath, and as I did, I was overcome by her love. I began to cry, something that was quite new for me. In my family, men almost never cried. I felt embarrassed, and yet Susan was very accepting of my tears.*

> *After that we made love, and it was as if something had opened up inside me. A dam had broken. I wasn't stopping my tears and feelings any more. I felt like a young boy and also like a powerful lover.*
>
> ARI, 32, SALESMAN

MOVEMENT

When we are at home with, and can welcome, our natural impulses to move, feel and engage with life, we feel more alive and more whole.

Life pulsates. The nature of our essence, our aliveness, is constant vibration. When a baby is unhappy, he cries. He wails. When he is frustrated his whole body shows it. He hollers with his whole body. When he is happy he coos. His whole body shudders with pleasure as he sucks on his mother's breast.

If we weren't loved for who we were in our early development, and instead looked for acceptance through actions that pleased our parents or teachers, or if the expression of feelings and the enjoyment of our own genitals was scorned or forbidden, we learned to suppress our natural impulses towards life, pleasure and love. In developing a more 'socialised' exterior, we may come to regard the natural pulsation of life as dangerous, as it threatens our perceived identity. This will have consequences in many arenas, such as self-consciousness in free dancing, or embarrassment and shame in simply inhabiting our own body. We may be plagued by the need to 'get it right' and 'perform' in sex, rather than simply following our own pleasurable and loving feelings in relation to our partner. In other words, both the more subtle bodily vibrations of energy and our free-flowing expressive movements become inhibited.

By relearning to recognise and follow our spontaneous life-flow, we can release these restrictive patterns and reclaim the joy and magic of being truly ourselves in life and in love.

Movement in life

By reconnecting with your impulses and spontaneous movements, you can support the process of reconnection to your life-force, your essence. Here are some suggestions:

1. Free dance, following the impulses in your body, rather than set steps or ideas of looking good. This can help to free up natural expressive movement.
2. Try kundalini shaking (*see page 53*), which is an excellent way to remember your natural pulsation, as it already has a vibratory quality. It has the capacity to lead you easily and gently back to your truth.
3. Express anger by beating a cushion and shouting 'no' for five minutes, then sitting in silence for another five minutes. This is known as Osho's Anger Meditation.

1. WITH YOUR BACK STRAIGHT, BREATHE IN AND RAISE YOUR ARMS ABOVE YOUR HEAD. BREATHE OUT, COME FORWARD FROM THE HIPS, AND SHOUT 'NO' AS YOU BEAT THE CUSHION.

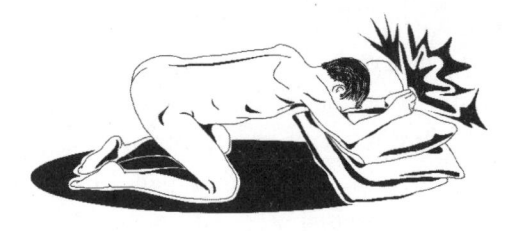

2. SIT IN SILENCE.

4. Let the playful child within you direct your movements. Have a 'playful inner child' afternoon with your partner or a friend. Take turns in deciding how to play together. Your inner child may like to dress up, play in the bath, play in the park or whatever takes your fancy!

> *Dancing as a meditation, I lost all sense of time, and became totally absorbed in the pleasure of movement, of freely expressing myself, just for me. The best way that I can describe the experience is to say that it was ecstatic.*
>
> LINDA, 42, CIVIL SERVANT

Movement in sex

As you make love, see if you can allow any spontaneous movements or pulsations that arise in your body to take place. Relax, breathe and follow your impulses. Be attentive in each moment to how your body wants to move, and in what positions it would like to be, to maximise your pleasure and enjoyment. How does your body want to express the sensations that you are feeling? Imagine your body as a piece of seaweed, soft, fluid and undulating, flowing in the tides of sexual energy. Follow the waves. Let your jaw be relaxed, and breathe naturally through your mouth.

Pelvic rocking meditation

This meditation can help you to find relaxed, pleasurable conscious movement in your pelvis. Pelvic rocking brings movement, blood flow and consciousness into your pelvis and supports this energy in expanding into the whole of your body.

The physical movement of pelvic rocking releases any tension stored in the lower back and lower abdomen, facilitating both a fuller and more integrated capacity for sexual passion. The rhythmic movement supports a more meditative attitude towards sexual pleasure, a 'relaxing into' it, rather than a 'need to do' something. By relaxing into a pleasurable experience, we allow it to deepen. A different, more diffuse and yet more holistic quality to the experience can then arise.

The Technique

Initially, practise pelvic rocking separately from lovemaking. You can then integrate any insights or discoveries into making love.

- Imagine that the horizontal line between your two hip bones forms an axle. Stand with your knees bent and legs apart. Rotate your hips forwards and backwards about this axle as shown in the picture (*see below*). Avoid any unnecessary movements in your upper body.

- Inhale as you rock your pelvis backwards (arching your lower back) and exhale as you rock your pelvis forwards (flattening your lower back). Relax and sink naturally into this rhythmic motion.

- Now, as you inhale and rock your pelvis back, also squeeze your pelvic floor muscles (*see page 116*). As you exhale and rock your pelvis forwards, release and relax your love muscle.

- You can imagine that you are breathing in and out through your pelvic floor.

- Continue for about five minutes, settling in to this rhythmic motion. Become aware of any sensations or feelings that arise in your pelvis and in the whole of you as you do this.

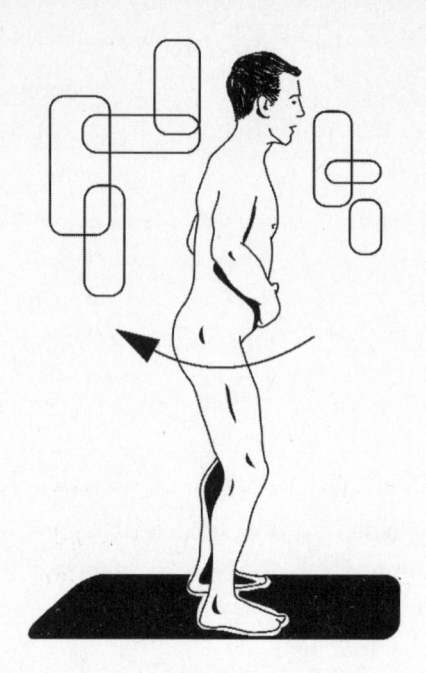

1. INHALE AND ROTATE YOUR PELVIS BACKWARDS

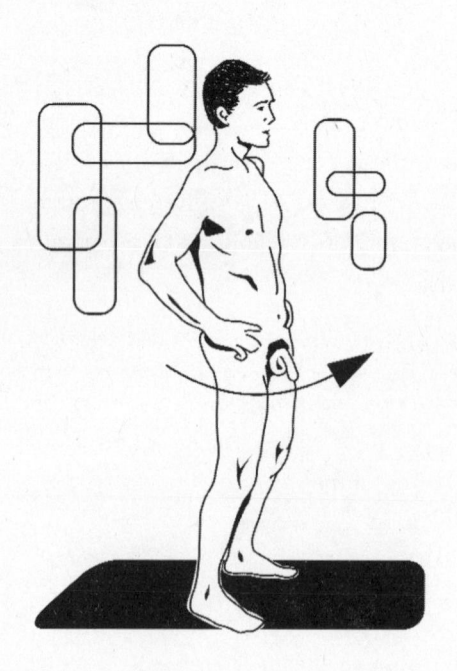

2. EXHALE AND ROTATE YOUR PELVIS FORWARD

SOUND

Utilising our voice to communicate our truth, needs, desires and delights in sex allows us to relax more and to experience greater satisfaction, bliss and ecstasy. The degree to which we can truthfully express ourselves with sounds and words in the microcosm of sexual relating usually reflects the ease with which we can communicate our true feelings, needs, wants and desires in the macrocosm of life. This correspondingly relates to our overall experience of nourishment and fulfilment.

Sound in life: expressive sound meditation

How easy do you find it to make spontaneous sounds? How do you feel about making a noise or saying what you really think and feel? What are the sounds and expressions that you would like to make if you weren't censoring yourself? Try this short exercise.

The Technique

This meditation will take about fifteen minutes. Play some recorded music that does not have words. Choose a vibrant, expressive piece, and play it as loud as feels comfortable. Put it on repeat, or else choose an album where the tracks have a consistent theme.

- Let the music encourage you to make sounds, in the safety of the knowledge that you will not be heard (much) above the sound of the music. Open your throat and experiment with guttural sounds. Do not attempt to be tuneful!

- Try some grunts and moans and yodels.

- Experiment with some higher-pitched sounds like baby noises, operatic singing, screeches and screams.

- Playfully make sounds with different emotional tones. Start with delight. Pretend that you are blissfully happy and want to tell the whole world. Tell them in sounds, rather than words. See if there's a spark of genuine exuberance or delight within you that you could give voice to.

- Express sadness. Experiment with sad sounds and notice where a moment of genuine sadness creeps in.

- Move on to anger.

- Then fear.

- Then back to delight again.

- Spend about two minutes on each stage, and when you are complete, turn off the music and sit or lie down in silence for five minutes. Notice any body sensations or feelings within you. Notice your response to the silence. Listen to the silence.

Sound in sex

When you make love, play with making sounds. Let the sounds that you make reflect the feelings and sensations in your body. Open your throat and see what comes out!

To become more aware of, and to practise communicating your needs, wants and desires verbally with a partner, go to the exercise on page 163.

Another intimate communication meditation involves making love and keeping talking all the way through. Let your voice continue an ongoing monologue of how you are feeling and what you are thinking. Don't worry about pausing to listen to your partner speak. Just keep going, even if you are both talking together. Say everything that comes into your mind, whether it makes sense or not. Do not censor anything. When you have finished making love, take some time to share how you feel and what this meditation was like for you.

RELAXATION

The final principle is relaxation. It is common to equate sexual tension with sexual pleasure. It is, however, absolutely possible and far, far more fulfilling to relax totally during the heights of passion. This allows pleasure to expand into bliss and ecstasy. In the whole of life too, as we relax, life's simple pleasures take on more brilliance, and moments of pain pass more quickly.

Relaxation in life

What, in life, makes you tense? Perhaps it's being held up in a traffic jam when you're already late, or having to be assertive and appropriately confront someone at work? Whatever it is that winds you up, you can moderate and modulate the effects of outside stimuli on your body by becoming acutely aware of the physical, emotional and psychological factors that are evoked in you. Do you clench your jaw and tighten your buttocks? Do you hold your breath? Do you imagine saying all sorts of obscenities from behind your locked teeth?

It's unlikely that having shoulders in your ears is going to help you face your boss or get the car in front of you to go any faster, so you might as well move some lactic acid out of your muscles and generate a few endorphins instead. Whenever you are tense, consciously squeeze the tight muscles while holding your breath. Then let go and exhale with a sigh.

Notice what you'd like to be saying to the person or people with you, or what you'd like to be complaining about to an imaginary friend or to God. Take a deep breath and, if there's nobody around, say it in gibberish. If there are others around and you wish to preserve your credibility, just breathe and imagine saying all the things you'd really like to be saying right now.

Sense how you are feeling, and how you are viewing yourself at this moment. Become keenly interested in yourself. Watch and observe, rather than analysing and thinking. As you become fascinated by your inner workings, witnessing this process, you are entering into meditation, and already you have a wider, more expansive perspective on life.

Relaxation in sex

While making love, do a quick body scan, from head to toe. Notice if your face is holding any tension. Take a deep breath, and let go of it as you exhale. Let your awareness work its way down your neck, shoulders, arms, torso, pelvis and legs, breathing deeply and letting go of any tension in your body as you exhale. Then bring your awareness to your genitals, vajra or yoni. Notice if you are at all tense here, or in the muscles around your sex organs. As you exhale, relax and let go. Continue for a few more breaths. You may be surprised to find that still deeper relaxation is possible as you continue breathing and letting go. Notice how this relaxation affects the sensations, feelings and experiences in vajra or yoni, and in the whole of your body.

> *I was surprised to find that as I relaxed my yoni more and more, I felt more, not less. I had generally been quite tense during sex, and getting aroused seemed to bring me even more tension! This was a whole different move. I was imagining relaxing yoni in bands, or rings, from the outside in, and found that I could really sense subtle tensions and effect a change in me. I became aware of pleasant sensations in yoni. She felt soft and juicy, and the warmth spread into the whole of my pelvis, and then twinkled in little spurts up to my head. My partner was also relaxing his vajra. That made a big difference, as I wasn't frightened that any minute he'd come and I'd be left hanging. I felt quite exhilarated afterwards, even though the experience itself had been very gentle.*
>
> Julie, 47, Massage Therapist

KEYS TO EXPANSION

Whether you're making love, at work or doing the shopping, you're likely to have a deeper experience if you allow yourself to become more expansive. Awareness is like a torch of consciousness, bringing light to dark places; clear intent is a note you sing to life so that life can hum in harmony; breath is a stream that can smooth and wash through our contracted patterns of thought and emotion, transporting us to the sea of energy flow; movement can crack the brittle shell of constricted expression, letting the phoenix rise from the ashes and spread her wings; as we liberate our voice we scream and sigh, moan and celebrate with the wind; as we relax, we sink down into the womb of mother earth. As we embrace who we really are, in each moment, as human beings, we join the dance of life.

CHAPTER SEVEN

THE CHAKRA SYSTEM

In Chapter 4 we explored the theme of becoming our own beloved, of learning how to enjoy and nourish the king and queen within. Chapter 5 showed the potential of intimate relationship to reflect back to us our beauty and our pain. Chapter 6 demonstrated the use of awareness, intent, breath, movement, sound and relaxation to 'open up' frozen parts of ourselves, to find more joyful and harmonious possibilities in sex and in life. In this chapter we develop these themes in the context of the energy centres in the body, the chakras. The chakras offer us both a route map and a direct line to healing and integrating ourselves, our sexuality, love and divine potential.

As the physical body is formed from the bones, muscles, organs, blood, nerves and hormones, in a similar fashion the energy body is structured by means of the 'chakras'. These are seven energy centres that govern different qualities of being and are intimately related to our physical structure and functioning. Together they form our 'energetic architecture'.

The Sanskrit word *chakra* literally means 'wheel'. We can think of the chakras as vortexes of energy, which interact with each other and the outside world. This chapter describes the qualities and roles of each of these energy centres, their locations and physical correlates, as well as their combined functioning. You can use this information as a springboard into exploring your own reality by doing the exercises and meditations in Chapter 8.

CHAKRA HEALTH

The 'health' of our chakras reflects the health of our bodies, emotions and minds. The seven chakras, located in vertical succession, incorporate the whole of the physical body. The ideal in Tantra is for all seven

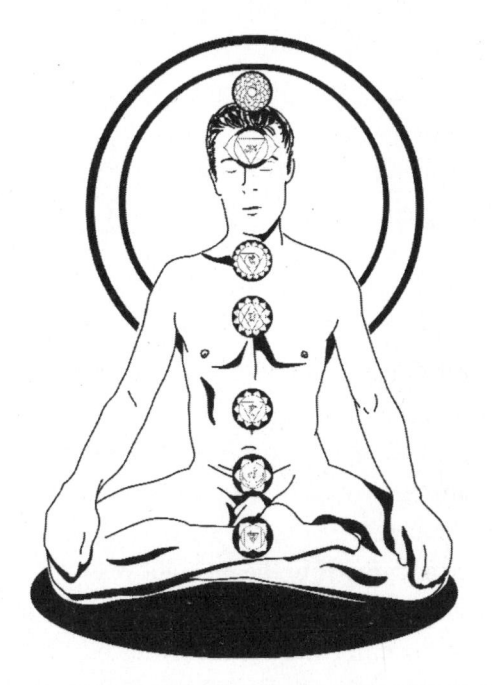

THE CHAKRAS FORM A STRAIGHT LINE DOWN THE BODY FROM THE TOP OF THE HEAD TO THE PERINEUM

chakras to be functioning at full capacity, so that we are able to clearly and with integrity celebrate being both fully human and simultaneously essentially spirit. When we make love with all our chakras in balance, Tantric Union happens.

The full energetic functioning of the chakras becomes unbalanced through the impact of non-optimal to severely traumatic life events, in particular those that occur in our early years. These life events encompass very early situations, such as the relationship between our parents when we were conceived, and the health and well-being of our mother during pregnancy and her attitude towards and connection with us in utero – all of them influence our energetic make-up and alignment. Then of course there's birth, childhood and the rest of life to contend with! No wonder most of us have a bit of healing to do.

To give an example, as our sexuality forms the ground of our being, a child who has been sexually abused will generally suffer consequences on many levels. As she has suffered a severe disregard of her natural boundaries, she may find it difficult in later life to assert appropriate boundaries and to know that she will be respected. The abuse may leave 'holes' in her energy field, representing a weakness and vulnerability in those areas. For example, she may have a hole in the third chakra, which is concerned with saying 'no' and preserving our integrity.

A healthy chakra maintains the capacity to open and close in appropriate accordance with will and the circumstances of each moment. In general, it is 'open' and available for engaging energetically with the world, and becomes more closed only when this is the most appropriate method of protection. Tantric chakra meditations can help to restore optimum chakra functioning. As we take a look at each of the chakras in turn, you will get a sense of the unique qualities of each one, and you will be able to begin to sense yourself in terms of your chakras and chakra health.

Each chakra also blends into the ones above and below it. They are all connected by means of a central channel called the 'inner flute'. You can imagine your torso, from base to crown, to be a hollow shoot of bamboo, like a flute, and the chakras are the notes through which the flautist expresses the divine melody of existence. In creating the soundtrack of our everyday lives, most if not all of the chakras are generally involved in how we interact with other people and our environment, and in how we see ourselves.

The Locations, Colours and Qualities of the Chakras			
CHAKRA	LOCATION	COLOUR	QUALITIES
Base	Perineum	Red	Life-force, rootedness
Second	Between pubic bone and navel	Orange	Sexuality, creativity
Third	Solar plexus	Yellow	Identity, boundaries
Fourth	Heart	Green	Love
Fifth	Throat	Blue	Expression, alignment with divine will
Sixth	Between eyebrows	Purple	Insight, clarity, intuition
Seventh	Crown	White	Essence, spirit, universal truth

THE FIRST CHAKRA

The first chakra, *Muladhara*, meaning 'root', encompasses the physical areas of the feet, legs and pelvis. It is associated with the adrenal glands, and is connected to our immune system. Its central point is the perineum, mid-way between the genitals and the anus in the pelvic floor. This chakra faces down, towards the ground. The qualities associated with it are our connection to and 'rootedness' in our basic life-force energy, our sense of safety and security in physical form, our connection with our 'tribe' or social context. People with healthy and open first chakras have access to a great deal of raw energy. They enjoy being alive, and trust that they will be provided for. Those with more closed or otherwise disrupted first chakras live in a state of constriction and anxiety. They fear that their basic needs may not be met, and feel somehow out of place in the environment in which they live. The colour associated with this chakra is red.

Case study

Karen, aged thirty-nine, a marketing consultant and mother came to see me because she wanted to rediscover her sexual fire and passion. She wanted to know orgasmic bliss and to experience her earthiness as a woman. I started by teaching her the Heaven and Earth meditation, where she was invited to become like a tree, with her branches reaching up to the sky and her roots reaching down into the earth. Reaching up to the sky with her branches felt blissful for her and gave her a sense of deep peace. She was naturally quite a spiritual woman, and had felt guided by Spirit most of her life. Reaching down into the earth with her roots, though, was more difficult for her. She kept getting distracted. It was as if part of her was saying 'no'. She realised that there was a bit of her that just didn't want to be here in physical form. She wanted to find her earthy passion, and yet in another way couldn't stand the thought of being human.

Karen's story is in no way unusual. In my work with the Tantric journey of connecting sexuality, love and spirituality, I find that many people, more frequently women than men, are already highly developed in terms of love and spiritual connectedness. Their challenge, then, is to integrate sexuality and their basic life-force energy into the picture. This inevitably involves making friends with the more raw emotions of anger and fear. When they feel safe enough to first experience and then surrender into these feelings, in a secure and appropriate setting, this also opens the door for them to let go into orgasm, and to reconnect once more with their true essence, which is at once both earthly and transcendent.

In almost equal proportion, there are on the other hand those (more commonly men than women) whose sexual energy and life-force are flowing pretty well, but who have a block in the solar plexus and/or at the heart. In other words, their first chakras are quite open and available. For these people, their 'direction of integration' with Tantra will be upwards, unifying their life-force and creative sexuality with a true sense of identity and the vulnerability of an open heart.

THE SECOND CHAKRA

The second chakra, *Svadisthana*, the 'seat of life', encompasses the physical region of the lower abdomen and lower back. It includes the bladder and kidneys, and is associated with the uterus and ovaries in women and the prostate gland and testes in men. This chakra runs laterally through the body, with its central location mid-way between the pubic bone and the navel on the front of the body, and the top of the sacrum at the back. The qualities associated with this chakra are those of our creative sexual energy and our 'gut instincts'. At the level of the womb in women, this is the place from where new life can grow and develop. It is our centre of creativity on all levels. In men, it is the place of the 'magical womb', an energetic mirror of the physical womb in women, with similar qualities to a woman's womb aside from the ability to incubate babies. It is the chakra concerned with one-to-one relationships and our human, relational expression of sexuality.

When this chakra is relatively closed or impaired, our creativity and sexual expression will be impaired. Women may have painful periods. Men may have prostate or ejaculatory problems. Both sexes are likely to experience relational difficulties. A person in whom this chakra is in a healthy state of openness is likely to have a full and healthy relationship with their own sexuality as well as with a partner. The colour associated with this chakra is orange.

Case study

Veronica was sixty-one when I met her. She had breast cancer with spinal metastases. She wanted to get in touch with her sexuality and her full womanliness before she died. I was moved by her willingness and courage. She was married, but had never felt fulfilled in her sexual relationship with her husband or with any of her boyfriends previously. She had mothered two children, whom she and her husband had adopted as babies since they had been unable to conceive. Her grief at feeling 'not a proper woman' was immense. On her first contact with the voice of her second chakra, her womb centre, she was able to release some of the grief, hopelessness and anger that had been held in this place. To her joy and amazement, the next time that she did the meditation her second chakra told her that her work was complete. Her womb said that it was her full and feminine womb, the deep mothering instinct within her, which had guided her in raising her two daughters.

Veronica's journey into her own sexual fulfilment was also beginning. At first she had no idea what she wanted sexually, so asking for it was out of the question. Her womb again had some ideas, as did her yoni and heart, and slowly she began to explore communicating her desire for a different way of making love (slower, with more cuddling, whole-body and genital stroking, and eye contact and verbal interaction) with her husband. Although challenged at first, he readily embraced the possibility of being able to eventually please his wife sexually, and in the process found that he was initiated into some of the ways of woman.

THE THIRD CHAKRA

The third chakra, *Manipura*, the power chakra or 'inner sun', centres around the solar plexus in the front and the mid-back around the area of the twelfth thoracic and first lumbar vertebrae. It encompasses the physical regions of the diaphragm, lower ribs, organs of the stomach, pancreas, spleen, liver, gallbladder and small intestine. It is the place from which we recognise our individual identity as separate from the social context, or 'tribe', in which we live. It is the centre responsible for maintaining our appropriate boundaries, for our 'yes' and 'no'. It is a reflection of our self-esteem, and as such it reflects our capacity to manifest our unique gifts in the world. It is the place of our 'charisma'.

People in whom this chakra is relatively closed or weak may have difficulty in asserting themselves. They may or may not know what they want in life, but even if they do they can encounter obstacles in acting upon their desires. The archetype of someone who says 'no' when she means 'yes', and 'yes' when she means 'no' falls into this category. Sometimes a person will compensate for a weakness in this chakra and become pushy and bullying. Since the third chakra is situated between the sexual centre (second chakra) and heart centre (fourth chakra), a constriction here will mean a lack of connection between love and sex.

When someone with an open third chakra enters a room you are likely to notice their presence. They may have a kind of radiance about them, and are likely to know what they like and want, and to be confident and forthright about getting it. The colour associated with this chakra is yellow, like the golden rays of the sun.

Case study

Caroline, aged thirty-one, came to see me for just two sessions. She wanted some help with asserting her boundaries, and to understand what she was 'doing wrong'. Caroline had been sexually abused by her father as a young girl, and had spent many years in counselling and therapy as a result. As a result of much inner work, she was now, for the first time, really in contact with her libido. She had a new boyfriend, and for the most part was very happy. However, whenever she went out to clubs or parties, or even while walking in the streets or travelling by public transport, she felt that men were looking at her inappropriately. Men she met socially would sometimes ask her out, even though they knew she had a boyfriend, and would disregard her 'no' as if they hadn't heard her say it.

I taught Caroline a way to strengthen her third chakra, involving making a sound from her diaphragm and using one arm and leg to symbolise projecting energy out from this place. This exercise, 'Shah!' is described in more detail in Chapter 12 (*see page 179*). I asked her to imagine that one of the 'leery' men whom she was unwittingly attracting was standing in front of her. I asked her what she wanted to say to him. She answered, 'Go away!' but in a rather unconvincing, helpless tone of voice. Then I invited her to do the 'Shah!' exercise, which she repeated several times, each time becoming clearer, more centred and powerful in herself. When I then asked her what she wanted to say to this man, she told him to fuck off in no uncertain terms. When I asked if she felt that he'd got the message, she said yes. Then she began sobbing. She realised that that was what she had really wanted to communicate to her father when she was a young girl of seven or eight and started to abuse her. At the same time, she desperately wanted and needed his love, and was frightened of losing him completely. She now understood why she had been giving mixed messages to other men.

THE FOURTH CHAKRA

The fourth chakra, *Anahata*, the heart, is centred in the middle of the chest at the front and between the shoulder blades at the back, and is our centre of love. This chakra encompasses the physical heart, and the whole of the chest, lungs, upper back, arms and hands. The endocrine gland at this level is the thymus, in the centre of the chest. It is the middle place between the three 'lower' chakras, which are primarily concerned with 'me', and the three 'higher' chakras, which are oriented more towards the transpersonal. The heart can be seen as the alchemist's crucible that transforms the lead of earthly life into the gold of divine union. It is often said that all healing takes place through the heart. Pure love is a direct expression of our essence. It is what connects and unifies all people.

When the heart is closed, we feel a separation from others and from ourselves. We think that by closing our hearts we can avoid getting hurt again (for it is past hurt that causes us to close the heart in the first place). This is true to a degree, since we feel love, loss and longing less keenly; however, this 'loss of heart' is itself a painful condition. Unresolved grief may play a large part in the development of heart and lung disease. When we 'harden our heart' we also increase the risk of hurting others by our words and deeds, like the proverbial bull in the china shop.

History and mythology abound with individuals who allowed their hearts to remain open amid even the greatest tragedies. Mahatma Ghandi and the Dalia Lama are but two of the best known of these figures, and there have undoubtedly been – and are – countless other beings of uncompromising love who have not received widespread recognition. Ram Dass, an inspired modern mystic, cites the story of a Tibetan monk from the time when China was invading Tibet, destroying monasteries and massacring monks and nuns. All the other inhabitants of the monastery had fled, and only he remained. When the most feared tyrannical Chinese warlord stormed the monastery, he encountered the monk standing alone before him. 'Do you know who I am?' asked the warlord. 'I could ram my sword through your guts without blinking an eye.' 'And do you know who I am?' asked the monk. 'I could have you ram your sword through my guts without blinking an eye.' The monk's love for humanity, truth and integrity, his compassion and deep inner peace enabled him to peacefully confront his aggressor in this way.

On a more everyday level, when our hearts are open we can give and receive love without an agenda. We may soar high on the wings of love, celebrating love's joys, and we are willing to risk facing our pain. We may experience compassion (being with others in their pain) and we become more fully human (humane).

And when [love's] wings enfold you yield to him,
Though the sword hidden among his pinions may wound you.

KHALIL GIBRAN, *THE PROPHET*

The colour of the heart chakra is green in most chakra systems (pink in others).

THE FIFTH CHAKRA

The fifth chakra, *Visuddha*, meaning 'purification', is about communication and sound, and is located in the throat and neck, the central axis running from the throat in the front to the occiput in the back of the head. It extends roughly from the collarbones to the top of the mouth, and includes the thyroid and parathyroid glands. This chakra is also connected with the will, and with harmonising our personal wants, desires and drives with our higher purpose in life, with 'Divine will'.

When this chakra is closed, we have difficulty in communicating truly. Words and feelings may get 'stuck in our throat'. Some people develop chronic or recurrent coughs or sore throats. A restricted fifth chakra may also indicate the suppression of a calling, for example to work with disadvantaged children, when that would entail giving up a financially secure job.

When this chakra is more open, the vocal quality is fuller and more resonant. There is greater congruency between what we mean and what we say, and we can allow fuller feelings to move through us as there is greater access to deep sobbing during grief, the force of anger, and also the sighs and moans of pleasure, and the blissful cries of ecstasy during lovemaking. Personal will is in better alignment and communication with a more receptive attitude of openness to being 'guided' by life. The colour of this chakra is blue.

Case study

Aldo grew up in a very strict Italian family where what his father said went, and he was not to answer back. Home life was so bad that at the age of sixteen he not only left home but also left the country. Whereas he built a good life for himself in Britain, at the age of twenty-nine he had still not had a long-term girlfriend. He came to Tantra to find out why, and hopefully to meet someone with whom he could establish a fulfilling relationship. I was struck by the little coughing sound that he made, as if something was stuck in his throat, whenever he spoke out loud in a group, or when he had something intimate or emotional to say. He too was aware of this cough, and told me how difficult he found it to speak out, as in his childhood he had been severely punished for doing so. Despite his impressive size and build, his voice was very soft, without much intonation.

It was not long before Aldo and Bettina, an effervescent, feisty and mature woman, got together. Bettina usually had something to say, and very eloquently at that. It became customary for her to speak for both of them.

Some time later, at another group, having done some healing work on reclaiming his masculinity, Aldo began to cough. He said that he realised that since being with Bettina he had let her take the lead, and that for the good of both of them it was time he asserted himself more and took up a bit more space. He said that from now on he was going to be more proactive verbally, both in his relationship with Bettina and in the workshop. It was clear that it involved enormous effort for him to put himself forward in this way. As he relaxed more into his flow, however, the coughing ceased, and the clearer, stronger voice of a courageous man who knew what he wanted and would not be held back by his fears emerged.

THE SIXTH CHAKRA

The sixth chakra, *Ajna*, known as the 'third eye', means 'to perceive' and 'to command'. This implies that when our perceptual capacities are more fully developed, we are in greater command of our lives. The chakra is located between the eyebrows in the forehead, and at the apex of the occipital lobe of the head at the back. It is the 'eye that looks inwards', our meditative and self-reflective capacity. It is the centre of intuition, clarity, insight and bliss. It is a sense of knowing beyond the logical mind. The pineal gland is situated here.

When the sixth chakra is closed we rely too much on logic. We can become 'stuck in a rut' in our ways of seeing the world, and may find difficulty in clearly making certain types of personal life decision. When our third eye is open, we have greater access to inspiration, a sense of spaciousness in the mind and a sense of rightness. When the third eye is open, and there is a clear connection between the sexual centre and this place, we can experience sexual arousal as a blissful sense of aliveness and spaciousness in the brain. The colour associated with this chakra is purple.

Case study

Retired publisher Evelyn, aged sixty-five, recounted to me what happened when she and her partner went away to Crete, on a week-long Tantra holiday. After a couple of days they found to their surprise and considerable dismay that they had both lost their desire. They talked about this in the group and the teacher said that it was just that the energy had shifted location, and asked them where it was now. He asked them to sit facing each other. They were instantly aware that the energy was at that moment, for each of them, in the sixth chakra, and they moved so that their third eyes came together. They stayed joined there for several minutes, and it felt totally appropriate and peaceful. There was a prolonged sense of openness at that place, of a different seeing.

THE SEVENTH CHAKRA

The seventh chakra, or crown chakra, *Sahasrara*, meaning 'thousand-fold', symbolising a thousand-petalled lotus reaching up to infinity, is situated at the top of the head. It includes the upper part of the head and extends several centimetres above the head. It opens upwards towards the heavens, and you can imagine this chakra as our direct link to God, to the Universe, the Great Mystery, or whatever for you is greater than your own individual identity. It is about the bigger picture. It controls the central nervous system function, and is associated with the pituitary gland, which is the control centre for most of the body's other endocrine functions.

People who are staunch atheists often have a closed seventh chakra. In these people, the degree of emotion associated with their conviction of an absence of God indicates an unresolved conflict with life. When someone suffers any kind of trauma, for example, and feels somehow betrayed by his idea of a benevolent God, he may feel powerless and resentful. The same thing may happen if, as a child, you had a natural sense of connectedness with the Divine, or qualities of deep sensitivity and perception. If your spiritual tendencies threatened the adults around you, you may have been ignored, chastised or ridiculed when speaking of such matters, so you learned to cut off from them in order to be loved and to survive.

When the seventh chakra is open, there may be a sense of living in prayer, of being loved by God, of trusting in the process of the unfoldment of life. Whether at peak moments of meditation, exercise, lovemaking or at any other time, you have a sense of wordless peace or ecstasy (going beyond your normal perceptual viewpoint); or whether you have an everyday trust in the unfolding of the mysteries of life, this is your seventh chakra opening. The colour of the seventh chakra is white, the brilliant white light of truth, which is the sum total of all the other colours of the rainbow.

Case study

Rob, a restaurant manager aged fifty-seven, said that after two previous occasions of doing the chakra breathing meditation (*see page 118*), he was becoming increasingly angry and frustrated. He resented some of the other people in the group who appeared to be having some kind of transcendental experience. So, the next time round, he decided to follow the advice of 'fake it till you make it'. He made a big deal of raising his hands to the sky and making ecstatic-sounding noises, while imagining white light raining down into him. To start with, he admitted that he felt a sort of 'fuck you' inside him. He wanted to make fun of all this crazy mumbo jumbo, as he saw it. Then, to his surprise, he did feel something coming down into him. He couldn't quite describe it, but it made him laugh outrageously, and then cry. When talking to some friends afterwards, he recalled instances from his childhood experiences in a very strict Catholic boys' school, where beatings for almost no reason were the norm. It made him wonder if somehow his anger at those teachers and priests had also caused him to block off believing in God.

This story illustrates the beginning of Rob's healing of his sense of separation from Spirit, which he had previously equated with the trappings of religion and the concept of a punitive God. Having a direct experience of something greater than himself opened him up to the possibility of the 'Great Mystery', and with it greater meaning and a sense of connectedness in his life. He became more open to seeing the essence in others, and eventually in himself, as well as to trusting the process of life more fully.

Now let's turn to the question of how to make contact with, heal and harmonise your own chakras, and how to allow them to open in such a way as to offer you a gateway to new worlds.

CHAPTER EIGHT

MEETING YOUR CHAKRAS

In the Native American tradition it is understood that we can benefit by receiving information with our minds, but that true change requires us also to engage the will of our spirit, to release and share our feelings and emotions, and to assimilate change in our bodies. Meeting and rebalancing our chakras offers us an opportunity to access our intuition and feelings, and through these our true will, by directly experiencing how we structure the energy in our bodies. This chapter focuses on getting to know our own chakras, and potentially meeting those of a partner. Chapter 9 progresses to the energetic exchange between lovers, and how to maximise fulfilment in lovemaking.

MEETING YOUR LOVE MUSCLE

In Tantra the muscles of your pelvic floor, those that encapsulate your genitals and anus, are called your 'love muscle'. If you are peeing and stop in mid-flow, you will use these muscles. This physical part of your anatomy is intimately connected with the energetic reality of your first chakra. In Tantra, the emphasis is not just on building up a strong love muscle, it is more about getting to know the feeling sense of this place in you, of building a relationship with it, from the inside. In doing so, you can not only vastly increase your genital sensitivity, and so your capacity to enjoy sex, but also develop a deeper and more connected experience of yourself and life as a whole. The topic of the love muscle is potentially huge and fascinating, and we explore it in more depth in workshops. Below is a simple introduction to sensing your love muscle.

The Technique

- Lie down on your back with your knees raised and feet flat on the floor.
- Relax and take some deep breaths.
- As you inhale, gently squeeze your love muscle. As you exhale, relax this area completely.
- Continue with this breathing/squeezing/relaxing cycle for roughly ten more breaths, noticing any sensations, feelings or impressions in your pelvic floor, vajra or yoni, and in the whole of you.
- Let go of the squeezing, and simply breathe naturally, again noticing how you and your pelvic region feel.
- Write down your experiences.

There is no right or wrong way to feel in this exercise. The most important thing is to be honest about what you are actually feeling, even if that's 'nothing'. In general, people's experiences range from nothing, which I call numbness, to discomfort, to gentle pleasure, warm pulsations and whole-body orgasmic experiences. If you embrace whatever you feel with curiosity, you will move more swiftly towards realising your potential in this area. This is because by being curious about whatever arises, you are developing a compassionate relationship with yourself and your sexuality. The less-pleasant experiences reflect your first chakra history, and the choices you made in yourself to deal with them. Your love muscle may be either weak from lack of practice or lack of 'presence' in this area (energetic withdrawal due to pain or shame), or it may be overly tight, contracted through fear of life or sex. As you become aware of and accept whatever arises, healing and balance and a relaxed engagement with your pelvic floor begins. The potential for deeper aliveness and great pleasure grows.

CHAKRA BREATHING MEDITATION

This meditation allows you to connect more deeply with a feeling sense of each of the seven chakras in turn through awareness, breathing, movement and sound.

It is a relatively 'yang' chakra meditation, meaning that it's quite active, with an emphasis on clearing out and reawakening the chakras. Its particular benefit is its capacity to get to the point without beating about the bush. It can really give your energy body a good spring cleaning, bringing held and rigid physical, emotional and mental patterns to the surface and supporting you to let them go. After doing the chakra breathing meditation you will often feel lighter, clearer, more in touch with yourself and more energised.

The real challenge in this meditation, as in most aspects of Tantric practice, is that the more you are 'total', entering fully into the experience, the more you are likely to feel. We all want blissful union with our own essence, our beloved and the Universe, but most of us want the roses without the thorns. Many of us are not willing to face our own fears, tears and less-than-pretty parts in order to discover the luminous still waters of our innate beauty that await us just below the turbulent waves of emotion above. It is impossible to open our hearts to love without also embracing the tears of our unfulfilled longings and heartbreaks. At this stage we do not need to understand what we are feeling or why we are feeling what we feel; we should simply allow these feelings to move through us, as we continue to return our attention to the meditation.

Our natural state of being is a vulnerable, alive pulsation. On top of that pulsation we erect protective walls in the form of physical tension, mental rigidity and emotional stagnation. I remember myself, as a workshop participant, doing the chakra breathing meditation, and feeling like a baby kitten afterwards; slightly wobbly, wide-eyed, alive, loving, soft and open. I couldn't imagine going about my ordinary life in this state, at the mercy of all the world's hungry dogs, and I was grateful to know that I could reinstate my walls whenever I chose to. I had imagined that being 'aligned' within myself would feel different from this, more solid, yet it was a relief to be able to let go of the hard edges that normally separated me from others and from myself, too, and I was able to enjoy a very deep sense of peacefulness, joy and wonder.

The Technique

The meditation can be practised alone or with a partner. The full meditation takes one hour, and involves three 'rounds' of chakra breathing followed by silence. The simplest way to participate in the meditation is to use the CD *Chakra Breathing* (*see* Resources, *page 250*), which guides you through the different stages with different pieces of music for each chakra, and bell chimes every two minutes to indicate when it is time to move from one chakra to the next. If you don't have the CD, play a continuous piece of wordless dance music and put it on repeat. Set a timer, musical alarm clock or mobile phone to ring every two minutes, or alternatively move on to the next chakra whenever you see fit to do so.

Grounding

- Whether alone or with a partner, begin with a namaste.

- Each stand with some space around you, eyes closed, knees bent and feet firmly planted on the floor, about shoulder-width apart. Feel the sensations of your feet touching the ground.

- Imagine that your feet have roots, reaching down into the earth. As you breathe, imagine these roots reaching all the way down, effortlessly, naturally and joyfully through the soil, the rock underneath the soil, all the way down to the molten lava at the core of the earth.

- As your roots contact this molten lava, this hot red fire of the earth, safely, effortlessly and joyfully, you can imagine this lifeblood of the earth to be your own hot red life-force energy, your desire to be alive in this body, on this planet here and now.

- As you breathe, imagine drawing this hot red life-force energy up through your roots, all the way up to the soles of your feet. As you sense, feel or imagine this hot red fire of the earth, of your own life-force energy at the soles of your feet, you can continue to breathe and draw this energy up into your feet and legs and into your pelvis.

Round 1

- Turn on the *Chakra Breathing* CD, or the music that you have chosen with a timer to chime every two minutes if possible.

Meeting your chakras — 119

- Continue breathing the red life-force energy into your pelvis. Remember all the qualities of the base chakra: a connection with the earth, with our sense of rootedness, family, connectedness. It is our foundation, and essential, primordial life-force energy, our passion for and trust in the experience of aliveness in this body, on this planet, here and now. It is concerned with meeting our basic needs. It is that animal drive for survival.

- Imagine now that you are breathing in and out through your base chakra at your pelvic floor. Breathe in and out through your mouth quite vigorously, but in a relaxed and effortless way.

- Move your pelvis any way that you like in time with your breath, to enhance the sense that you are breathing in and out from that place. The breathing sounds on the *Chakra Breathing* CD are quite fast. Some people find that they end up trying hard to keep up and feeling stressed in the process. There is a bit of an art to being able to move and breath quite fast and energetically, and yet to remain relaxed. I would therefore recommend that you start by finding your own natural breathing rhythm, even if that is relatively slow. From here, gradually experiment with speeding up your movements and breath, while staying relaxed. If you notice that you are tensing up, return to the slower rhythm.

- Focus on the inhalation, filling your body with breath. Simply relax on the exhalation. You may sigh, or have that letting-go feeling of sighing. Do not push or blow the air out with force, as this can lead to hyperventilation. Simply let it flow out of you naturally, without controlling it in any way.

- You may like to touch your perineum to help your awareness settle in that place.

- As you exhale, experiment now and then with making some sounds that relate to your experiences of your base chakra at that moment. If you feel pleasure, you can moan. If you feel irritated or angry you can growl. If you have no sense at all of your base chakra, 'fake it till you make it', as Margot Anand, one of my teachers, says, and play around with some sounds. See which ones resonate with you, increasing your sense of aliveness or realness, as you do this. Many of us, particularly if we are British, can find it difficult to make spontaneous sounds. We can feel embarrassed lest we appear silly, or in case we get it wrong. The great thing about spontaneous expression, however, is that you can't get it wrong! The more you put in, the more you'll get out of it, so you might as well go the whole way!

- Notice any feelings or body sensations that arise in you as you do this. Allow these feelings or sensations to be here, perhaps even exaggerate them and express them with your voice, as you continue to relax your body as completely as possible (while still standing up!) and breathe into your base chakra. Be open to any spontaneous images or impressions that emerge as you breathe into your base chakra.

- After two minutes, a bell will ring on the CD and the music will change slightly. If you are using other music without a timer, move on when you sense a connection with your base chakra.

- At this point, move your attention up to your second chakra, between your pubic bone and navel, the centre of your creativity and sexuality. Imagine that you are breathing into your second chakra as you move and undulate your body, especially focusing on your lower abdomen and lower back, the area of your second chakra. You may like to visualise the colour of the second chakra, which is orange, if you find that helpful. Continue as for the base chakra with breathing, movement, visualisation, sound and awareness, noticing any feelings, body sensations, images or impressions that arise as you do this.

- After another two minutes, another bell will sound. It is now time to progress to your third chakra. Again, repeat the process, now breathing into your third chakra, and from here, every two minutes, move up to the next chakra, all the way up to your crown.

- A summary of the locations, colours and qualities of the chakras is given on page 103.

- At your crown, you may wish to raise your arms in the air as a gesture of receiving from above.

- After two minutes at the crown, three bells will sound on the CD. You will then have two minutes to let your attention descend through each of the chakras down to the base, allowing the white light of spirit/essence/truth to merge with and infuse all the other chakras, bringing the qualities of spaciousness, healing and peace, until you arrive back at your base. This is the completion of the first 'round' of chakra breathing.

Rounds 2 and 3

- If you are doing the meditation alone, rounds two and three are the same as round one. Simply repeat the process. Each repetition will take you deeper into your chakras and support them in opening to their full potential.

- If you are with a partner, for the second round of chakra breathing, sit comfortably back to back to each other, both cross-legged. Do not talk during the meditation – just find your way into this position together.

- Repeat the process of breathing into each chakra, from base to crown, and then merging the qualities of the crown with the other chakras as you come down, as before.

- As you sit back to back, breathe, move, make sounds and feel, you will inevitably be affected by your partner. This is an amazing and challenging opportunity for you to take responsibility for your reactions to your beloved.

- If your responses are of pleasure and connectedness, great! Enjoy! If, however, you are becoming irritated with your partner, perhaps because they're moving too much or making too many loud sounds, or maybe because they're not moving at all or giving you any sense that they're even alive back there, notice your own responses. Resist the temptation to blame your partner for how and who they are, and instead let yourself feel more deeply what is evoked in you.

- By taking responsibility for your own feelings, you can learn and grow from the experience, with gratitude towards your partner for being your mirror and showing you more clearly parts of yourself that may be causing you pain, and giving you opportunities to transform your belief systems and behaviour patterns.

- For the third round, if you are with a partner, you can lie down in a front-to-front cuddle, or sit together in the posture of 'yab-yum' (*see page 244*), breathing through your chakras as before in whatever form of connection you choose.

Silence

- Three rounds of chakra breathing, whether alone or as a couple, are followed by the final stage of silence. This stage is far more than a 'rest break', and neither is it a 'think break'; it is an integral part of the meditation. If you are in yab-yum, you may wish to move into a more easily comfortably sustainable position together. Then simply sit or lie together in silence, relaxing into whatever you sense or feel in your body. Any time that your mind wanders, simply bring it gently back to the present moment: your body, your breath, sensations and feelings in your body.

- There is no right or wrong way to feel. As you relax in awareness and stillness and presence, a natural integration of the process of chakra breathing can occur within you.

- If you are usuing the CD, a bell will sound after fifteen minutes. This is the end of the meditation. Complete with a namaste.

- If you are with a partner, take a few minutes each to share your experiences of the meditation.

I'd always felt a bit distrustful of people who could have orgasmic experiences simply through breathing and imagining something. I didn't know if there was something fabulous out there that I was missing out on, and if I was in some way inadequate, or whether those people were either nutty or faking it. So when Gemma and I had an amazing experience doing the chakra breathing, it really took me by surprise. It was the third round, and we were lying together, breathing into our hearts. Suddenly it was as if our two hearts were wafting together, merging into one. I can't really describe it, aside from that it was a light form of ecstasy, an

> *amazing spiritual orgasm. We were going 'Oh God! This is amazing!' without words. Neither of us wanted to move on, it was just so blissful.*
>
> CARL AND GEMMA, 37 AND 36, ADVERTISING DIRECTOR AND MARKETING MANAGER

CHAKRA TALK

This meditation helps you to get to know the 'personality' of each of your chakras, through letting them speak. Bear in mind when doing the exercise that not all of your chakras may be immediately ready to communicate with you, particularly if they harbour very old, painful memories. Treat yourself with compassion and gentleness. Let the chakras that are ready to speak share with you, and be patient with those that aren't. In their own time they will open up.

The Technique

The meditation can be done alone or with a partner. If you are alone, you will need either a tape recorder or a pen and paper. You will need about ten to twenty minutes per chakra. In each session of chakra talk, you will hear the voice of just one chakra at a time. You may repeat the exercise for another chakra, on the same occasion, but it's best not to engage with too many chakras at once, as this can dilute the experience of the uniqueness of each chakra. It is generally best to start with the first chakra and progress upwards in sequence with each session of chakra talk.

- Take a little time to enter sacred space and share a namaste with yourself or each other.

- Sit comfortably upright. If you are with a partner, sit opposite them. Decide who will go first, and which chakra will speak.

- Place your own hands on the central area of that chakra on your body. Feel the contact and warmth of your hands. Imagine that you are breathing in and out from that chakra, noticing any sensations, feelings or awarenesses that arise as you do this.

- In your own time, when you feel that your attention has settled in the chakra, begin to talk (or write, if you are on your own, and prefer not to use a tape recorder) as that chakra, beginning with the words: 'I am [*your name*]'s first [*or whichever chakra is speaking*] chakra.' For example, if my second chakra was speaking, I'd begin with: 'I am Leora's second chakra …'

- Then let your chakra continue to speak in the first person about its reality as that chakra. This may appear odd at first, but soon you'll discover that each of your chakras actually has a separate voice, an individual quality like a personality, and a reality that is slightly (or extremely) different from what you ordinarily regard as yours.

- Some subjects to invite your chakra to speak about might be:

    How it is now.

    Its history through your life.

    Its pain and regrets.

    Its joys and unique gifts.

    Its longings.

    Its relationship and connection with other parts of you.

    The essence, the universal qualities of this chakra.

    Any special messages it has for any people in your life, present or absent, alive or dead.

    Any special messages it has for you.

- When your chakra has finished speaking, take a few moments to silently, or out loud, thank that chakra for sharing its reality with you.

- Slowly take your hands away from the contact with your chakra, and let your awareness return to the whole of you. Notice how you feel now, having heard your chakra speak.

- Complete the experience with another namaste.

- If you are with your partner, you can spend a few minutes sharing with them the implications of what your chakra has said, and how you may incorporate these insights into your life. If you are alone, you can similarly spend a few minutes writing down or contemplating this theme.

Dave, at thirty-five, described his life as 'beige'. He didn't feel things strongly any more, and had lost his drive towards intimacy and sex. He wanted to discover the life and feelings within him, his passion, and his sense of fun. He wanted to learn how to establish deeper connections with others, and how to love. Dave was very reticent before the chakra talk meditation, thinking that nothing would happen for him. To his great surprise, when his heart chakra communicated directly with him, this strong-willed, quite tough-looking man found himself in tears, as his heart revealed its tenderness. He said, 'I was amazed. Absolutely. An incredible release and a beautiful experience I never knew could exist. It was as if my heart was truly speaking.'

Like Dave, you can let yourself be surprised! Being curious is a wonderful approach to Tantra, as you may have completely different experiences of these meditations each time you practise them. I recommend practising each of the meditations at least twice before moving on to the next chapter, which will guide you deeper into your sexual-loving potential as a man or woman, for yourself and in connection with your beloved.

CHAPTER NINE

MALE AND FEMALE ENERGY FLOW

We have now explored the theme of becoming full and whole in ourselves, and energetic principles and practices that show us how to do that. This chapter is specifically devoted to the differences between being a whole and fulfilled woman, and being a whole and fulfilled man, in energetic terms. Here I invite you to explore energetic exchange as love partners, the basis for open-hearted, fulfilling lovemaking.

In my early twenties, I'd reached an impasse regarding men and sex. It seemed that if I fell in love with a man, he wanted first to have sex with me, and after that he'd consider opening up to love. But I wanted to know that a man loved me before I would open to him sexually. I remember talking to a girlfriend and marvelling at how men and women ever got it together, since it seemed that we were at best such different creatures, at worst incompatible.

I wanted men to be more like women, and yet I ended up pretending to be more like a man. I changed my rhythm and pushed myself to have sex even when it wasn't with the whole of my being, in order to get love. And then I wondered why I wasn't fulfilled.

Many of the men I meet, both socially and professionally, speak of a similar, though complementary dilemma. Women these days, they say, expect a 'New Age', loving, caring and considerate man – one who will look after the children, wash up, listen deeply and talk about his feelings. When it comes to bedtime, they want a 'heartful warrior', a powerful, sexual, potent male with the heart of a Buddha. 'I just can't do it!' the men lament.

So if women are trying to be more like men, and men are attempting to become more similar to women, and it's still not working, maybe there's another way. Tantra suggests that by entering deeply into our feminine nature, as a woman, or our masculine nature, as a man, we can find a sense of harmony and fulfilment within ourselves, our own natural flow. From this place, man and woman can meet and join in love and sex with deep mutual connectedness, in a spirit of celebration. It's about finding our true, mature, vulnerable and yet strong, integrated masculinity and femininity.

MALE AND FEMALE ENERGY FLOW

I begin by describing our energetic potential as men and women, and ways in which we may move away from this energetic alignment. Thereafter, in the following section, I introduce you to an exercise to re-establish sexual-loving flow and fulfilment.

When a man's energetic flow is congruent with his physical and energetic potential as a man, that is, when he is in harmony with himself, then he is positively charged in his sex. Positively charged means that he is ready to interact with the world from that place. A man's genitals protrude from his body as a physical reflection of this energetic state of readiness. Correspondingly, he is negatively charged, that is receptive, in his heart.

The male energy flow

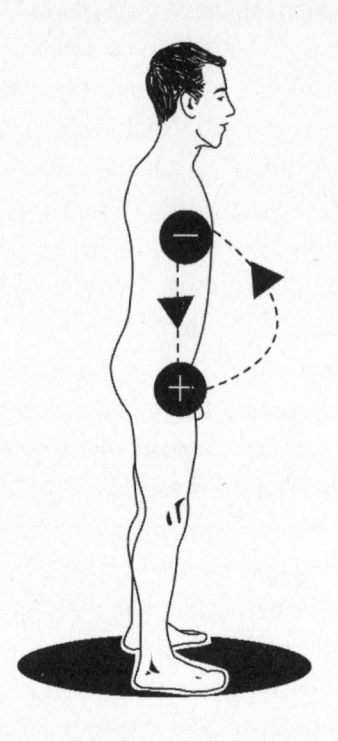

These two poles, positive and negative, active and receptive, form an inner battery, as shown in the drawing (*see above*). Inside his body, there is a flow from negative to positive. The love in his heart flows down into his sex, so that he is genuinely sharing his love in offering his sex. Outside his body, there is a flow from positive to negative. He receives his sexuality, his desire to share his love and sexuality, in his heart. He welcomes and celebrates his masculine sexuality. He is self-contained, not requiring another to be complete, and yet available for open sharing of himself with others and his beloved.

The above description is of a man's potential. In real life, many men are not in touch with and do not live in this male flow of energy. For some, it is simply a matter of knowing that the potential offered by the male breath is available. Once they have the knowledge and the physical-energetic experience in their bodies, it can be one of those sudden illuminating 'aha!' moments.

In other men, there has been a disruption of the natural flow between heart and sex, as a result of childhood factors such as the sexual relationship between their parents, and how their sexuality was received when they were young or when they were growing up. The relational and social circumstances in adulthood, such as those already mentioned, may also contribute.

Ben's early life events obstructed his innate male flow. His energy habits are the best possible compensations that he could find, given his experiences, and the resources he had available to himself at the time.

Ben is a loving man. He gives a lot of love and support to his partner and other people in his life. He is a good listener. In bed, however, things are different. Ben is either very horny, or hardly interested at all. Either way, his sexuality lives a relatively separate life from his heart. After sex with his partner, he has a tendency to roll over and go to sleep. He sometimes enjoys pornography, which is a form of safe sex, sex without relationship. Sex for him is about excitement and release. Love is something different. Ben loves one woman, but is attracted to someone else. This is because he holds a huge amount of tension in his diaphragm, which prevents any love descending into his genitals or sexuality from rising to his heart. He is literally split, heart and sex.

When Ben was a young boy and started to play with his willy, his mother told him to stop in shocked and no uncertain terms, and said that it was disgusting to do that. She also told him that willys were dirty. So Ben, as a young boy and later in adolescence, touched himself only in secret, and with a considerable degree of shame and guilt. When, in adult life, he loved a woman, he couldn't equate love with sex, as sex was dirty and love was pure. He felt somehow seedy when he was being sexual with a woman he loved. He was ashamed of admitting his sexual needs and desires, and consequently found it difficult to relate to hers. If a lover ever said 'no' to a sexual advance, he felt immensely rejected. He wanted a woman to unconditionally love and accept his sexuality in the way his mother hadn't. He was extremely confused in himself about how to be with his own sexuality, and underneath the confusion both deeply hurt and enraged by his mother's rejection of this essential aspect of his being. Whenever Ben now feels rejected by a partner, he becomes angry with her and distances himself from her in order not to face the awful feelings of worthlessness and rage that rejection evoke in him.

Ben is not the way he is by any accident. He learned these ways of being in response to childhood experiences that did not model or recognise what it was to be an integrated man.

Let us look now at Mike's account of healing his relationship with his masculinity. Mike grew up in an environment where he associated masculinity with macho-ness. The men in his life as he was growing up, his only role models for masculinity, were overbearing and aggressive. Women were frequently regarded as objects for men's gratification. Tenderness and vulnerability were seen as signs of being effeminate. Not altogether surprisingly, Mike did not aspire to be a powerful, sexual man (as he saw it to be then).

Mike's rejection of the images of masculinity he grew up with left him with a big gap in his identity. He felt ashamed of his masculinity, and frequently experienced difficulties in maintaining erections. This re-enforced his self-image of inadequacy.

Through Tantra, Mike has become more comfortable with his sensitive, feeling side, has learned to cry and has found that his partner actually sees his capacity to share vulnerability as a sign of strength rather than weakness. Through techniques such as the male breath (*see page 135*), he has learned to infuse sexuality with love, and to experience potent, male sexual loving. When he was in touch with this flow, his partner accepted him sexually whether he was erect or flaccid, and they found avenues to meaningful intimacy that did not depend on him having an erection. Paradoxically, with the pressure to perform and the dependence on erection for confirmation of his masculine potency removed, Mike found that he was having far more longer-lasting erections.

As a result of seeing his masculinity in a new light, in harmony with his softer, more receptive feminine side, Mike now feels far more comfortable, and in fact proud of being a (genuinely) powerful, sexual man.

Through practising the male breath, it is possible to 'rewire' yourself, to redirect your energy into a regenerating and rewarding flow.

The female energy flow

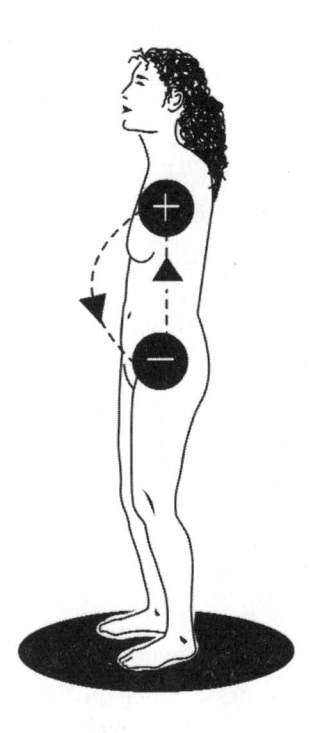

When a woman's energetic flow is congruent with her physical and energetic potential as a woman, that is, when she is in harmony with herself, then she is positively charged in her heart and thus ready to interact with others from here. A woman's breasts protrude from her body as a physical reflection of her energetic state of readiness. Her breasts also represent the erotic expression of her love. A woman is receptive or negatively charged in her vagina, or yoni.

A woman's positive and negative poles form a battery, as shown in the drawing (*see above*). Inside her body, there is a flow from negative to positive, from yoni to heart. The sexual charge in her yoni rises up to her heart, and she experiences the joy of sharing her heart that is also alive with her sexuality. Outside her body, she can receive the love she shares in her yoni, as she allows the penetrative love emerging from her heart to enter her yoni; she is once more replenished. She celebrates her own flow and potential. She is whole in herself and yet can further delight in sharing herself with her beloved.

Women who have been sexually abused, or who habitually have sex as a means to get love, may find it difficult to allow their yonis to be receptive. It is common to compensate for invasive sexual experiences either by becoming very tight and closed in yoni, or by entering into the male energy flow. It may be necessary to move through some of the original feelings associated with yoni in her receptive form, in order to embrace the beauty, magic and power of true receptivity in this place.

For me, learning the female energy flow and integrating it into sexual relating was a complete revelation. I discovered, for the first time, deep fulfilment in lovemaking. I felt as if my beloved's vajra was entering my yoni and extending right up to my heart. I felt truly loved. My yoni was wide open, relaxed and full of delicious aliveness. It brought tears of joy to my eyes.

It is this receptivity in yoni, and the flow from yoni to heart, that determines the difference between giving from the heart, from fullness, which is a natural, joyful overflowing, and giving in order to get, or giving from emptiness, which gives rise to resentment and burnout.

THE MALE AND FEMALE BREATH

Through breathing with intention, moving, making physical, emotional and energetic contact with our own bodies, sex and heart, we can open the way to returning to harmony, within ourselves and with our beloved.

The male breath

The male breath is best practised when the body is warmed up and fluid, for instance after kundalini shaking (*see page 53*). If possible, spend about fifteen minutes shaking, and while your body is still vibrating, begin the male breath.

> ### *The Technique*
>
> Continue to play the music that you have used for kundalini shaking, if you like, or any other wordless, repetitive and rhythmic upbeat music, at relatively low volume. You may like to remove your clothes – being naked can help you to connect more deeply with the experience. You can take anything from ten to thirty minutes each time you practise the male breath.
>
> - Stand upright with your knees loose and gently vibrating.
>
> - Place a hand on your heart, and the other hand on your vajra, your sex.
>
> - With your eyes closed, breathe first into the hand on your heart, feeling, sensing, seeing, hearing or imagining your heart chakra beneath your hand. Imagine that your hand is cradling your heart. Take a moment to sense or feel, to listen or allow images to arise from your heart, noticing what is present in your heart at this moment. Simply acknowledge and welcome whatever you find.
>
> - Then do the same with your sex, tuning in to what is present in your vajra at this moment, again welcoming whatever is here.
>
> - Once you have received both your heart and sex, as you exhale, stroke down your body from your heart to your vajra. Imagine that you are breathing the love from your heart into your genitals.

- As you continue to exhale, imagine that you are breathing out of your vajra, sharing your love-infused, penetrative sexual energy.

- Let your hand movements represent the direction and intention of your energy flow, so as you exhale, let your hands sweep out from your vajra. Notice what happens inside you as you do this. Then let your hands loop upwards so that as you inhale, you receive your sexuality in your heart. It's as if you're delighting in your own sexual flow and sexual expression. As you exhale, again stroke down your body from heart to sex.

- Continue to breathe and stroke and move your hands in this way, connecting with the intent and meaning of what you are doing, while sensing what happens inside yourself as you do this. Let your body be alive, vibrating, fluid and in motion.

- It can be helpful and may add to your enjoyment to sway or thrust your pelvis forwards in a fucking movement as you exhale from vajra, swinging your pelvis back as you inhale.

- Allow what is happening within you to guide your body movements, hand expressions, and so on. Let the whole of you be responsive to the moment, being with what is actually happening inside you, rather than what you might like to be feeling or experiencing.

- When you are ready to complete, simply let go of the hand movements and stand, relaxed and in silence, noticing any feelings or sensations within you. Open your eyes when you are ready.

When you are able to let go into the sensations and subtle feelings in your body, you may experience a flow of love and sexual feelings, a sense of strength and softness, joy or an impression of coming home, as the following account shows.

> *As I engaged with the male breath for the first time, I soon felt a very physical sensation of movement inside, something trickling down from my heart to my balls. It was almost like being stroked on the inside. Every time I breathed in, I felt my heart was getting bigger and bigger as I felt more and more love coming in. When I breathed out and down into my sex, I could feel all that fullness dropping into my balls. It was so sexy! As I breathed out from vajra, moving my pelvis in a fucking motion, I had a delicious, almost orgasmic feeling. It was completely amazing, feeling all this love becoming sexiness, and then sexiness becoming love again.*
>
> *Since then, it's felt like a doorway has opened. A doorway that I didn't know was there before. Now I can access that feeling any time I like. The experience showed me how to trust and let go into my body. Now lovemaking is entirely different. I just let go and my body just does it! I don't need to think or plan or try as I did before, which I now realise was coming from my head. I feel far more in touch with my love, and feel it coming out through my vajra.*
>
> Roger, 55, Holistic Doctor

The female breath

Begin as with the male breath, with fifteen minutes of kundalini shaking (*see page 53*). This will warm up your body, help you become more present, and awaken movement and energy flow inside you. Another option is to spend fifteen to twenty minutes dancing quite vigorously or jumping up and down.

The Technique

Take about ten to thirty minutes to enter into the female breath. Have some energetic, wordless music playing at low volume in the background, and if possible remove your clothes. Close your eyes, and while your body is still in gentle motion or vibration, staying loose and soft in your knees, begin the female breath.

- Place one hand on your heart and the other on yoni.

- Imagine that you are breathing in and out of your heart, cradling your heart with your hand, and take a few moments to sense, feel, imagine or see how your heart is at this moment. Notice if it is open or closed, happy or sad, frightened or jubilant. Simply acknowledge whatever is present in your heart. Then bring your attention to yoni.

- Imagine that you are breathing in and out of yoni, cradling her with your hand, and again take a few moments to sense, feel, imagine or see what is present in yoni right now. Again, simply acknowledge whatever you find.

- Now, as you inhale, draw your breath up from yoni to your heart, stroking with your hands on your body in accordance with your breath. Breathe the juiciness, the sexiness in yoni, up to your heart. Notice whatever you feel, sense, see or become aware of as you do this.

- Allow your heart to be filled, then, as you exhale, imagine that you are expressing the love that is in your heart. Let the gesture of your hands reflect this expression.

- As you inhale again, loop your hands down to yoni, and receive in yoni the love you have for her, the penetrative, expressive love in your heart.

- Continue with this cycle, noticing how you feel as you do so.
- Let your body remain in gentle, fluid motion, undulation or vibration. Let your pelvis, torso and neck be relaxed and mobile. Let these movements be a natural expression of what is happening inside you, rather than any formulaic recipe.
- Let your breath, movement, feelings and experience be alive and spontaneous in each moment. Let it be as it is, rather than how you might like it to be or how you think it should be.
- When you are ready to complete the female breath, let go of the hand movements and rest for a few moments in silence, sensing and feeling your body. Open your eyes when you are ready.

Here is an account of how one woman experienced the female breath.

> *I felt, on my in-breath, a rising of phallic energy within my body. In one sense, it was as if my clitoris was extending up inside me. I have heard it said that a man wants to fuck a woman right up to her heart and mouth. Well, I felt as if this giant clitoris/penis was extending right through my heart, up to my mouth and beyond. I wanted it to completely move through me. My early history had predisposed me to feel great fear of men, and yet this experience of masculinity was altogether positive. It was as if the masculine and feminine components in myself were uniting, and this meeting of opposites was very exciting. It happened gradually, like a subtle ladder rising up inside me and supporting me. For me this was a pretty revolutionary step, as I had felt very little sexual desire for many years, and this feeling of sexuality was both new and yet very much internal.*
>
> CATHERINE, 54, GRANDMOTHER

What else you may feel

If you are not already living in the male or female flow, you may also encounter either body sensations or emotions that indicate where your energetic 'blocks' are. For example, you might notice a feeling of constriction in your solar plexus (or in your heart, belly or genitals!). As you continue with the male or female breath, this may become more noticeable, and may even become painful. Carry on with the male breath, but see how relaxed you can be as you do so. It may be that lying down on your back with your knees raised will help you to relax and let go. In this way you may find that the male breath melts away the constriction or pain that you feel.

Sometimes this melting will involve the release of emotion. This is the emotional content of the energy block, and it's generally best to simply let the emotion flow, and to leave trying to understand where it came from until afterwards. It is also possible that you will feel the emotional content of an energetic constriction immediately, without a concurrent body sensation. This is just as welcome. Again, let yourself express whatever you are feeling as you continue to breathe. Let the breath and your intention, awareness, relaxation, movement and expression open up the channel to your natural energetic flow.

As you challenge your formative experiences, you may also feel the impact that they have had on your body and in your life. Moreover, as you connect with the relief and joy of recognising your innate sexual-loving flow, you may feel the grief at having been out of touch with your naturalness for so long.

MALE AND FEMALE ENERGY EXCHANGE

Once you have practised your own flow and have become aware of your habitual energetic patterns or blockages, you can take responsibility for your experiences in relationships with others, your partner in particular. If, as a woman, you are fearful of allowing yoni to be truly receptive, and as a result you have been holding or clenching your love muscle very tightly, then it is unlikely that you will have been able to receive a partner fully in sex. In recognising this, you have the opportunity to release your partner from the onerous task of having to fulfil you sexually; you may now focus on allowing yourself to receive. The female breath can guide you.

If, as a man, you experience shame, fear or embarrassment in truly allowing your expression of sexuality from vajra, then you have a chance to free your beloved from having to be the one to make you feel like a real man. You can devote yourself instead to reclaiming your potent masculinity for yourself. As you enter into the male breath, you may find your virility waiting to flow through you.

If you are seeking that feeling of being in love, of the merging of love and sex, and you notice that your solar plexus and diaphragm are like a steel plate separating the upper and lower parts of your body, then finding another lover is not going to help you in the long term. The way forwards is to open to that inner marriage of your own love and sexuality.

Taking responsibility for ourselves can be daunting. It's much easier, sometimes, to blame our problems on our partner and to stay stuck. When we change ourselves, it can be like jumping off a cliff: we need to let go of our old ground, our old identity, to make way for the new. As we leap into the unknown, we can only trust that we will find our wings, and that they will carry us to a new land. If we knew in advance where we were heading, it would be easier to simply get on a plane and go there. Inner transformation, however, cannot give us advance guarantees. We often need to experience the freefall before we realise that we had wings all along. The good news is that others have taken the plunge before us, and they can vouch for the fact that it's worth it.

The male–female breath

The male and female breath, as well as offering us insights into our inner energetic reality, can support us in transforming the old into the new. As we continue to breathe in this way, we are rerouting our irrigation channels to allow in the waters of life.

Once you have come to know yourself and your flow, without needing to be whole, healed or perfect first, you are ready to allow an exchange with your partner. The male and female energy exchange is the energetic basis of lovemaking that allows love and sexuality to flow together within yourself and between you and your partner.

The Technique

This exercise takes about twenty minutes.

- Warm up your body with shaking, dancing or jumping, as before (*see page 135*), with your eyes closed.

- Remaining in relaxed motion, open your eyes and greet each other with a namaste.

- Close your eyes again, and for yourself enter into the male or female breath.

- When you feel connected with your own flow, open your eyes. Let your gaze be receptive, as you continue with your own breathing cycle, in eye contact, allowing yourself to be witnessed, and to allow your partner in.

- After a few minutes, become aware of your hand movements and breathing rhythm. *Staying in touch with your own flow*, gradually find a way to allow your two circles to become one as shown in the drawing (*see above*). You may like to imagine that your hands and those of your partner can feel each other through the air in between them, and they move together as one.

- Whoever is sharing from their positive pole (vajra for men, yoni for women) directs the speed and intensity of flow from that place. In other words:

- Men, as you breathe out from vajra, sharing your sexuality, you decide how fast or slow, how subtle or intense, is the energy you offer to your partner.

- Women, as you receive in yoni, receive what is actually given. Inhale and draw your hands in to yoni as your partner exhales and extends his hands. Let your rhythm and the intensity of your breath match his.

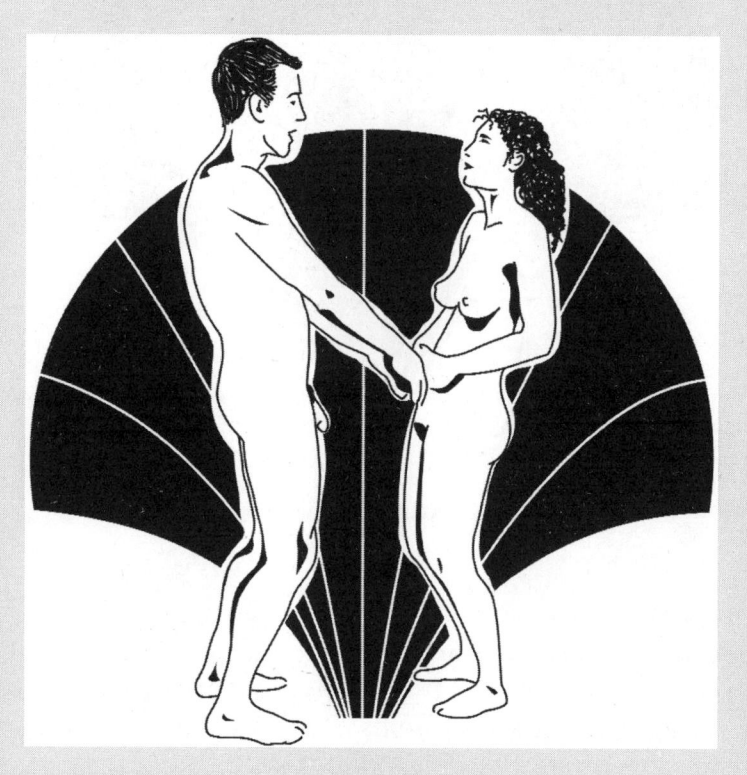

- Women, as you exhale, sharing the love from your heart, extending your hands towards your partner's heart, you lead. Men, you let the rhythm and intensity of your in-breath reflect those of your partner's out-breath. In this way you are genuinely receiving what she has to share with you.

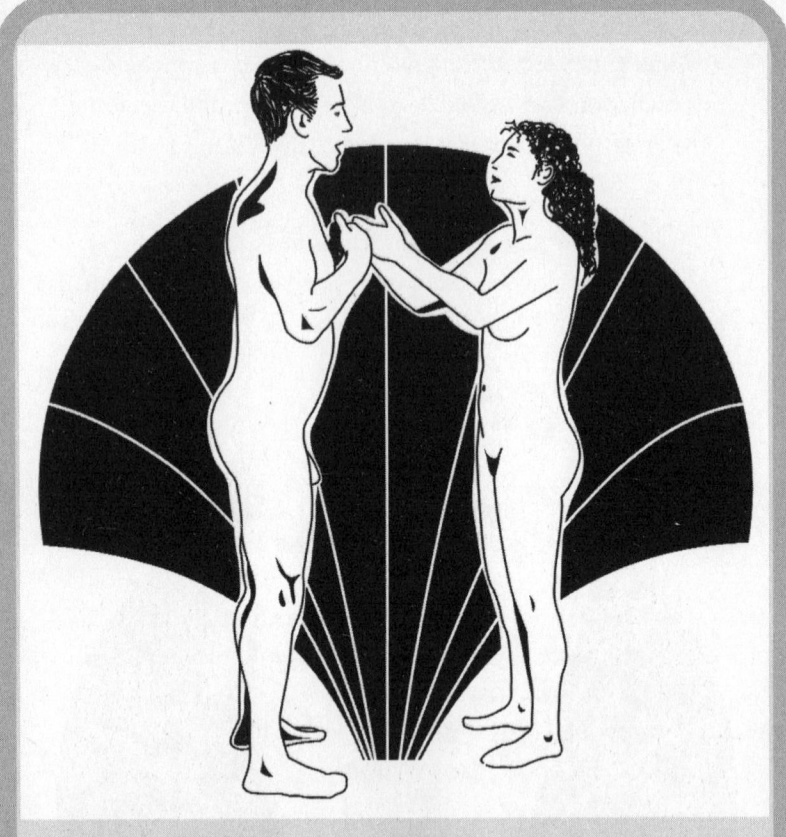

THE MALE AND FEMALE BREATH

It's a delicate balance, being present with your partner and in the exchange between you, and simultaneously present in yourself and your own flow. If at any time you sense that you have lost touch with yourself, simply close your eyes for a while until you have regained your sense of connectedness with yourself. The male-female breath is an energy building exchange. One gives while the other receives, and vice versa. It is this giving and receiving, combined with the inner flow between each partner's own sex and heart or heart and sex, which allows the love and passion to grow.

- You and your partner can sense the right moment to complete this exchange. Generally, it's good to stop once you have both felt a sense of connectedness and exchange. If this is not possible, return to your own flow, with your eyes closed, to re-establish your own relationship with yourself, before completing.

- When you are ready, let go of the hand movements, close your eyes and take a few breaths in silence, noticing how you feel.

- Thank and honour each other with a namaste.

- Take some time to share your experiences.

Doing the male breath while Gemma was doing the female breath, I had an experience that I couldn't have intellectualised. I was standing there, exaggerating the movements and breathing, and something took over. I felt myself expanding out. I really felt my balls, I felt really in touch with myself, powerful and strong, and yet still caring and in connection with Gemma. I think that up to that point I had been overly concerned with doing the exercise right and pleasing Gemma. I'm someone who doesn't get into an argument unless I'm really pushed to the edge. I like to be seen as nice and accommodating. When I was in my male flow, that stuff didn't matter to me. What really mattered was me being honest, real and passionately me, and that wasn't dependent on how Gemma responded.

CARL, 37, ADVERTISING DIRECTOR

We were Tantra novices and felt quite daunted when we turned up for our weekend course, but any fears were soon dispelled by the pervading atmosphere of love and warmth.

> *There is no doubt that all the exercises we did brought us closer together over the course of the weekend, but we both agreed that the male and female breathing was our most powerful experience. In working together, breathing in through the heart and out through the sex, we were left with an almost overwhelming feeling of sharing the same breath and love in a timeless circle of energy. It was amazing to feel so spiritually combined with another person. There were elements of erotic sensation, but the experience was much bigger than that word implies. Having said that, we did end up conceiving our third child during the weekend!*
>
> JULIAN AND POPPY, 43 AND 38, JOURNALIST AND RESEARCHER

SAME-SEX COUPLES AND OPPOSITE GENDER ENERGY FLOW

What I write here on the energetics of same-sex relationships comes from my experience of working with lesbian women and gay men, and from my experience and understanding of energetic principles. It is my perspective to date, and I do not claim it to be absolute truth!

My perspective is that, whatever our sexual preferences, we are a man or woman as defined by our physical sex first, and straight or gay second. Thus a lesbian woman is a woman first, lesbian second. Here we come to the topic of gender and identity. 'But I don't feel like a woman,' say some of my lesbian clients – yet neither do they feel like men.

There is a correspondence between how we 'run our energy' and our inner experience of masculinity and femininity, whatever our sexual preferences. A heterosexual woman can relate to her partner and the world from the position of the male energy flow and still be heterosexual. Similarly, a heterosexual man can 'flow' in the female energy cycle and still be straight. We can have access to both flows within us, depending on the circumstances and our choices.

In referring to same-sex couples, I shall now focus on lesbian lovers, as I have more direct experience in this area than I do in working with gay men. I hope that gay men can extrapolate, as corresponding energetic principles apply.

A lesbian woman who is in touch with her female energy flow knows what it is to be a woman. She can then, if she is able and inclined, also engage in the male energy flow. A lesbian woman who has no access to the female energy flow may well have a good sex life, if she is able to allow her energy to flow in the male cycle. She will, however, be less free to be sexually receptive in a way that includes her heart (a feature of the female energy flow).

In a couple where both women are in tune with the female energetic flow, to the exclusion of the male flow, their relationship can include a deep and fulfilling sharing of love and sexual intimacy, and this can last a lifetime. Their sexual relationship is unlikely, however, to be very passionate. Passion occurs when opposites meet, like the poles on a magnet.

I have not met a lesbian couple where both women were energetically in the male flow. My guess is that they are either not attracted to each other, or that these relationships do not last long, past the initial sexual excitement. I am open to discovering otherwise.

Where two same-sex lovers meet sexually and one is in the male flow, the other in the female flow, there can be love and passion, sex and relationship. If this flow is always in a certain direction, however, in other words if one female partner is always in the male energy flow, I am not sure if this will be ultimately completely fulfilling for her forever more. A woman knows, deep down, her potential for receptivity in sexuality, and her capacity to transform this into love. There is likely to be some irritation, some sense of loss at her separation from her full womanliness, somewhere down the line. My sense, therefore, would be that if both partners were grounded in their own-sex flow, and had access to the other-sex flow, there would be room for choice, creativity, fun, sharing, love and passion. The same is true for heterosexual women and men.

TRANSCENDING GENDER

In fact, some aspects of Tantra are ultimately about going beyond sexual and gender differences by blending the male and female flows within us. It seems, therefore, that either by gaining a deep appreciation of the essence of femininity (for a woman) or masculinity (for a man), or by melting and harmonising male and female principles within us, we can realise the unifying essence of all things. This requires that we first establish our identity, our separateness. Once we know who we are, we can begin to discover who we are not! In other words, according to Western spiritual teacher Ram Dass, we need to become a 'somebody', to know who we are in ourselves and in the world, before we can become a 'nobody', someone who transcends these distinctions. If we try to be a 'nobody' too early, we end up lost.

In my experience, however, many people, both homosexual and heterosexual, whether single or in couples, do not have access to either the male or female flow! In these cases, anywhere that is most easily accessible is a good starting point. Each time we give, we risk not being received. Whenever we open to receive, we may get hurt. Tantra in general, and the male and female energetic cycles in particular, are not easy. In entering into them, we risk opening ourselves up deeply, and need to have the resources to risk being hurt in order to fully love and to exchange our sexual gifts. This attitude to risk is eloquently summed up in the following well-known poem.

> *To love is to risk not being loved in return.*
> *To live is to risk dying.*
> *To hope is to risk despair.*
> *To try is to risk failure.*
> *But risks must be taken because the greater hazard in life is to risk nothing.*
> *A person who risks nothing, does nothing, has nothing and is nothing...*
> *Chained by his certitude, he is a slave, he has forfeited his freedom.*
> *Only a person who risks...*
> *Is free.*
>
> FROM THE POEM 'RISK', ANON

CHAPTER TEN

OPENING TO LOVE

This chapter is about loving ourselves exactly as we are, here and now in our bodies, as sexual beings. It is about letting go of whatever obscures this potential in us. It is about melting, letting our rigid exterior soften to reveal the tender, radiant being within. It is about allowing ourselves to feel.

Prerequisites to self-love are self-awareness and self-acceptance. As we become aware of ways in which we judge our own feelings and physical appearance, we can choose to let go of such attitudes, and open to new possibilities, as Mike's account, below, shows.

> *I realised that I had put a lid on my anger, and in doing that I had put a lid on everything, including my love. All my feelings flattened out and nothing really meant much to me any more. When I took the lid off my anger, having learned that it's OK to feel anger, and that anger itself isn't bad – it's what you do with it that counts – I started to feel everything.*

> *That's when I learned to cry, and to really laugh. And to love. Now, when my partner says she has something that she needs to talk to me about, I know that even if she says something that makes me feel uncomfortable, in the end, if I keep letting myself melt, our love and joy will deepen.*
>
> MIKE, 42, COMPUTER ANALYST

It isn't that we need to try to love more, because love is our essence, our true nature. But we do need to devote time, effort, clear intent and commitment to noticing, and to letting go of how we obscure the love in us, and the love that's available for us to receive from other people and other sources. When we allow ourselves to feel all our feelings with compassion and awareness, and without blaming anyone else, then we increase our capacity to feel and to heal, and hence our capacity to love.

BODY LOVE

Are your thighs too fat, or your muscles too small? Are you too hairy or too hairless? Is your hair too grey or too dark? Is your penis too small? Are your breasts too small? Or are they too large? Is your belly too big?

How we relate to our physical bodies reflects how we relate to ourselves. If the body is the temple of the spirit, we can't throw rotten eggs at its walls and expect its interior not to smell. We don't have to be our ideal shape and size, even if this is within the bounds of biological possibility, in order to love ourselves in our physicality. We can start now, and begin by noticing how, in fact, we do feel, think and behave towards ourselves, both outside and in, and to be open to receiving with compassion whatever we find. The body love meditation or ritual is a way in.

The body love ritual alone

The ultimate aim of this meditation is for you to transform how you relate to yourself.

The Technique

You will need about twenty to forty minutes, a full-length mirror, a notebook and a pen.

- Begin with a namaste, honouring yourself and your intention to explore the possibility of loving yourself and your body more.

- Stand, fully clothed, in front of a full-length mirror. Look at yourself up and down, and notice what thoughts and feelings, judgements and appreciations arise in you.

- Look yourself in the eyes, and receive yourself with your gaze. Spend a few minutes simply being with you.

- Begin to remove your clothing, one item at a time, being aware of what thoughts and feelings arise in you. Breathe comfortably and fully. Receive your eyes with your gaze at times. Carry on until you are naked, or until you have removed as much clothing as is right for you.

- Look at your body, and write down what you *don't* like about it and why.

- Look at your body, and write down what you *do* like about it. Notice what touches you about your body, what you find beautiful, handsome or moving about your body, what you are proud of and why.

- Take another look, and see if there's anything about how you are in your physicality that you may have forgotten to appreciate, or that could be seen in a different light. An example that springs to mind is a slim and petite friend of mine, who gave birth to twins. She has some loose skin over her lower belly now from the pregnancy, and initially she found this aspect of her body unattractive. However, she later realised that she was and is incredibly proud of all her children, and of her capacity to birth and mother twins. She began to see the loose skin on her belly as a mark of her femininity, maturity and wisdom, and of the joy that her children have brought her.

- Take some time to honour and celebrate your body. One popular way to do this is to have a loving shower or bath in honour of the Shiva (male aspect of the Divine) or Shakti (female aspect of the Divine) in you. Enjoy the sensations of the water caressing your skin, and afterwards take a few minutes to either rub some moisturising cream into your skin, or to gently caress or massage your own body. Notice how you feel as you do this. Write down in your notebook what your thoughts, feelings, body sensations and realisations have been.

- Complete with a namaste to the Shiva or Shakti in you.

If you have less time than suggested here but still want to devote regular time and energy to healing your body image, you can spend just five or ten minutes a day looking at yourself in the mirror, noticing what thoughts and feelings come up for you, and being open to being compassionate towards what you see in yourself. You can devote any bath or shower to being an honouring of the male or female in you, and you can spend five minutes afterwards either massaging cream or oil into your skin, or simply caressing or massaging your body.

It is good also to keep a diary of the thoughts and feelings that arise in you. It's a process of becoming more aware of how you treat yourself, and where you are hard or judgemental on yourself. This process is unlikely to be linear – there may be days when you are very unkind to yourself, and others when you feel at peace and very loving.

Body love ritual with friends

This is a more advanced version of the above, which is taught at intermediate Tantra workshops. At home, you will need to find two or more like-minded, same-sex friends. With witnesses, an added benefit is that you may discover that other people perceive you differently from how you perceive yourself. You may also notice if you tend to be far more critical towards yourself than you are towards others, and you will have a clear choice to see yourself in a new light.

The Technique

You will need about 45 minutes per person and, if possible, a sarong each. Explore this ritual in a warm, comfortable room where you will not be disturbed.

- Make a cosy nest of duvets, cushions and pillows large enough to be able to lie down in, preferably against a wall (for back support).

- Share a three-way (or four-way or five-way) namaste.

- Decide who will go first. I will refer to this person as 'number one'.

- Supporters, sit comfortably in the nest, giving your full attention to number one, who stands up in front of the nest.

- Supporters, whatever you are thinking or feeling, please do not speak until the stage of the ritual where you are invited to do so.

Opening to love — 153

- Number one, as you stand in front of the others, close your eyes and take some deep breaths. Notice how you feel. It is common to feel nervous receiving so much attention, when you are here to be honest and open, to reveal yourself more fully, rather than to perform. As you continue to breathe deeply and fully, open your eyes and receive the gaze of each of your companions. Allow any support, care, respect or love that you see in the eyes of your supporters to touch you.

- Throughout the ritual, continue to make eye contact with your friends at regular intervals, as well as to breathe and notice how you are feeling. If at any stage you have an impression of being not fully in your body, pause and see what you need to come back to the here and now. Having one of your supporters holding your hand or making physical contact in some way can often help.

- Next continue with the stages of the body love ritual described earlier, namely:

    o Removing your clothing, slowly and consciously, noticing how you feel. In this case, also communicate these feelings with your supporters, and periodically pause and take some deep breaths in silence, receiving their gaze. Remove as much clothing as is right for you at the time. It is better to leave some clothes on, and to feel present in yourself, than to take everything off if that means becoming so uncomfortable that 70 per cent of you has disappeared into the ground!

    o Showing and describing what you don't like about your body.

    o Showing and describing what you do like, and why. Include aspects of the whole of your body, for example your tallness or suppleness or voluptuousness.

- After that, stand silently, breathing, facing your supporters. It's their turn to tell you what it is that they find beautiful, attractive, handsome, moving, inspiring, pleasant or evocative in your physical body. Supporters, it is absolutely vital that you are honest here, and that you share from your heart. If you have nothing to say, say nothing. In my experience, it is rare not to be touched by the presence and beauty of another human being's body.

- Number one, don't discuss, dispute or deny what they have said. Simply listen, receive, breathe and notice how you respond. Notice if there are any ways in which you discount, distance or disregard what the supporters are saying. See if you can allow the supporters' words to touch you. I'd like to draw a distinction between appreciation and desire. Just because, supporters, you're enjoying looking at the body of another man or woman, does not mean that you've become a homosexual. Whatever your sexual orientation, it is possible to appreciate the beauty in someone without wanting or needing to be sexual with them.

- After giving feedback, supporters lay number one's sarong out in the nest, and invite him or her to sit or lie down on it. Number one, this is an opportunity for you to receive some loving contact from your supporters, for you. Perhaps you would like a hug, cuddle or massage, or to be gently caressed, or to receive some motionless touch or firm contact from the supporters, for example on a part of your body that is tense. You decide what you would like, from whom (it can be all of the supporters, or just one or two). If the supporters are able and willing to offer you the contact that you have asked for, you can go ahead and receive it, for about five to ten minutes.

> - When the contact stage is complete, supporters slowly and consciously remove your hands from number one's body. Number one, sit or lie with your eyes closed for a minute or two, feeling your body and skin and noticing how you feel inside.
>
> - When you open your eyes, take a few minutes to thank and acknowledge your supporters.
>
> - Let your supporters dress you (or if you prefer, you can dress yourself) in the clothes of the 'new you'. Your current new clothing is your sarong, but subsequently you can choose anything you like to represent any changes that have occurred in your self-image as a result of this ritual.
>
> - Number one then comes to sit in the nest, and it is the turn of number two.
>
> - After everyone's turn, complete with a group namaste, and take some time to share your experiences.

Once, when I was leading this ritual at a women's workshop, one of the participants was a stunningly beautiful, twenty-two-year-old model. Her experience of the body love ritual was quite poignant. It may not surprise you to hear that the other women in her group were acutely envious. They admitted later to have been thinking: 'Well, it's all right for her!' When it came to her turn, however, the model was sad and tearful. She said that she didn't feel seen, loved or appreciated for who she was. Men were attracted to her physical beauty, but she didn't really feel that they loved the real woman underneath. Women were often cold and distant towards her, out of jealousy, so she found it difficult to befriend women, as she was afraid of their resentment. Her honesty and vulnerability moved the other women, and opened the path for a two-way healing. The model was seen, accepted and embraced for who she really was, beyond her looks. The other women were able to see that the cultural ideal of physical attractiveness that they had been envious of isn't everything, and they were more able to accept their own unique brands of womanly beauty.

Duncan was in his mid-fifties when he did the body love ritual. Initially he found it difficult to say anything, until he recognised that he was cutting off from his feelings. He told his supporters how he felt embarrassed at being seen naked, it was just something one didn't do. As he continued, he found himself talking about his white chest and pubic hairs. He became immensely sad, and began to cry. He saw his white hairs as an irrevocable sign of ageing, ageing that he did not feel from the inside, but was apparent from the outside, 'a silent reminder of my mortality' he called them. When he finished crying, something changed in him. 'I felt passionately alive. Knowing that I was getting older gave me the impetus to bloody well get on and do something meaningful with my life.'

If you are part of a couple, you may be wondering why I'm not suggesting doing this with your partner. I would actually say that this is a beautiful ritual to share with your beloved, but only after you've done it at least once with others, or several times on your own. One woman who came to Tantra with her partner was terribly upset about her lack of self-esteem. Her partner adored her and told her how beautiful and talented she was on many occasions, but she couldn't let it in. She thought, 'Well, he would say that, wouldn't he!' After doing the body love ritual with women, however, everything changed. She really 'got it' that she was beautiful, and that the women in her nest were genuinely speaking from the heart, with no ulterior motives. Afterwards, she was able to allow in her partner's words of love and praise, and even decided to have a 'celebrating herself' day!

Another reason to do the ritual separately from your partner first is that some people who have been in a relationship for some time find that they have become dependent on their partners for their self-definition. Body love offers an entirely different perspective, in that it is about starting with you. If you allow your partner to define who you are, then you become like a leaf in the wind, skipping on the breeze if your partner is flattering, sullen on the damp ground if they are not. Remember, the Tantric ideal is to meet your beloved as a king or queen, whole and complete in yourself, coming together to share gifts and to celebrate. The body love ritual is a step in that direction.

Self-love beyond the body

The body love ritual is not just about our physicality; it's also about the body as the temple of the spirit, and as we take time to appreciate our temple, we inevitably invoke the presence of Spirit. On a purely human level, if we hate our body and judge ourselves for how it looks, it will be more difficult to delight in our inner beauty. When we forgive ourselves for not being physically 'perfect' as we imagine perfection to be, we open up the space to enjoy and celebrate our own unique brand of male or female form. As we accept and embrace our external looks, our self-esteem and appreciation of our inner landscape also expand.

The glue that attaches us to a poor body image and a negative view of ourselves is called shame. It is healthy to feel shame when we've done something that is anti-life, such as harming someone. This shame is related to the action we have taken that we now regret, and is healthy in that it supports us in feeling remorse, and hopefully making amends and not repeating this behaviour again. However, as has already been discussed, when we have been taught as infants, children, adolescents and adults that our bodies and sexuality are dirty and bad, then we end up believing that we ourselves, who are essentially physical sexual beings, are dirty and bad. This is toxic shame. It is not healthy. Toxic shame is anti-life.

As we now look upon our bodies, including our sexual organs, and allow ourselves to be witnessed, it is as if we are shaking out an old mattress, and all the dust that has been lurking inside comes to the surface. The mattress is becoming clean once more, but what we perceive is a cloud of dust. The waves of nervousness and embarrassment that we may feel in the process of disrobing and talking about our bodies is like the dust being dislodged from the mattress. If we breathe and stay present in our physical and emotional experience, we can allow these feelings of 'hot shame', which is toxic shame evaporating, to move through us and out of our systems. As we meet shame head on in this way, without getting lost in it or the belief systems that keep it lodged in place, by remaining in the here and now, in eye contact with our supporters or ourselves in the mirror, we become more and more shame-free. We are uprooting the weed of shame, leaving fertile soil for self-acceptance, self-esteem and self-love to flourish.

In contrast, when we try to bypass or override shame, we are simply trampling on the weed, which continues to grow underfoot. Because shame is stifling, oppressive and extremely painful to live with, it is natural to try to break free. Many people do this with alcohol, or uncharacteristic bouts of hedonism, where, for a while, all inhibitions are thrown to the wind. In shameless moments, it is tempting to go beyond our natural boundaries as a reaction to the repression we have been suffering. After several drinks at a party, you may find yourself doing and saying things that at the time give you that exhilarating sense of freedom, but in the morning shame returns tenfold as you ask yourself 'What have I done?' Sadly, this pattern of oscillating between shame and shameless and back to shame again has the long-term effect of reinforcing the hold shame has on our lives.

In order to be truly free, we must face the feelings of shame that have been organising our inner world in consciousness, and in conjunction with anchoring ourselves in the world of reality, the here and now of the body, and of relationships based on truth and love.

CHAPTER ELEVEN

OPENING TO PLEASURE

Pleasure is God's gift to life. Our basic life functions are modulated by pleasure and pain. As mammals, we humans are unusual in that our bodies are awakened to sexual pleasure, whether or not this is connected with potential conception. Could this mean that we are designed to make love and enjoy sexual pleasure?

Tantra is the ultimate form of hedonism, and yet it is totally different from what is commonly thought of as hedonism. Tantra is not about chasing pleasure out there, which requires more and more and greater and greater thrills to keep the juices flowing, but it is about maximising our capacity to open to and receive pleasure from the whole of life. It is about returning to sensitivity, and allowing the pleasure that we experience in our sense organs to expand into an experience of universal connectedness, of oneness. As the Tantric sutra goes:

> *When receiving a caress, Oh Princess, enter into it as everlasting life.*
>
> SHIVA SUTRA

By allowing ourselves to be fully present in each moment, to enter deeply into the simplest of sensory experiences, we can contact our essence, the Universe within. This is why Tantric texts describe the senses as the gateways to Spirit.

In order to be fully available to open into pleasure, we need to:

- Be able to feel and appreciate pleasure in our bodies.
- Know our boundaries, our edges, that is to know what is me and what is not me; what I want and what I don't want.
- Know that we are worth enough to have what we want.
- Be able to clearly express our choices.
- Relax, open and receive. To be fully present in each moment.

PLEASURABLE CHOICES

At the heart of Tantra is choice. Tantra is essentially about choosing to say 'yes' to life. And yet, until we are able to truly express our 'no', to know when we mean 'no', and to have that respected in relationships, then our 'yes' is not clear. We need to know that we have choice, and to recognise the choices that are available to us.

Choosing appropriate boundaries

Many people find it difficult to say 'no'. Others find it hard to hear a 'no' from someone else, because they experience it as rejection.

If your boundaries as a child were disregarded or abused, your capacity to say 'no' may be impaired. If it were a simple matter for us all to just say 'no' when we meant it, to know when we meant it, and to trust that our needs and preferences would be respected, we'd already be doing it. For many people, reclaiming our 'no' to what we do not want is a process that may be a prerequisite of genuinely opening up, to saying 'yes' to pleasure.

> *Saying 'no' did not fall naturally within my family. The messages I was given around my use of the word 'no' were that I was mean, selfish and only ever thinking of myself. I grew up with this belief.*
>
> *In relationships with men, and in sex, I veered between rigidly defining my position, what I do and don't do, almost before the subject had even been raised, and at other times going along with things I didn't want because of my desire to please, to be loved, to be sensual. It was a painful and confusing mess, and I pushed away many a potential loving mate through anxiety and confusion.*
>
> *Then, at a Tantra workshop, the issue arose again, with one of the male participants. I wanted to say 'no', but couldn't. My impulse was to run, but that wasn't the point. I knew that this was a chance to do something different. I could hardly speak, I felt sick, my head felt as if it was about to explode.*
>
> *Leora kept reminding me that I did have a choice, a choice to say 'no'. Finally, from somewhere I heard a tiny voice, my voice, saying 'no'. With each repetition, my voice got louder and louder, until finally it came from my heart. From my soul. 'No', 'No!', 'NO!'. No word had ever sounded so good.*
>
> *There has been a change in my life since this amazing experience. I am now less rigid in my 'no's, and in fact I'd say I more routinely say 'yes' to my life now. But when I feel a 'no', I express it, even when it's difficult.*
>
> AMARA, 41, LAWYER

At the other end of the line, if we habitually interpret someone else's 'no' as a rejection of who we are, we are in trouble. When our partner says 'no' to sex, we may immediately imagine that they no longer love us. Suddenly, whether sex happens or not that night becomes almost a matter of life or death. In reacting in this way, we miss the opportunity for genuine intimacy, for understanding more about our beloved and why sex does not appeal to them just at that moment.

Learning how to say and receive 'no', and still to remain in contact, in relationship with that person, with an open heart, hugely widens our potential for pleasure and intimacy.

'Yes, no, maybe and please' exercise

This exercise requires two people, either you and your love partner, or you and a friend. Your 'menu' of contact will be different depending on whom you are sharing the experience with. It need not be an erotic occasion, but it can be if the time and partner are right. For friends, a shoulder massage or a loving hug are pleasurable options; for lovers the world is your oyster!

There are two roles in this exercise, the 'Active Recipient' and the 'Initiator'. The role of the Initiator is to follow his or her impulses in relation to the Active Recipient, without words. The role of the Active Recipient is to give feedback to the Initiator, letting them know whether or not you are enjoying how they are interacting with you, moment by moment. The Initiator then responds to the feedback given.

The Technique

You need between forty-five minutes and one and a half hours in a place where you will not be disturbed. Some gentle background music may also be an asset.

Decide your roles. You will swap around, so it doesn't particularly matter who goes first. Decide also how long each turn will be. Something between ten minutes and thirty minutes is ideal.

- Share a namaste.

- The Initiator stands about three feet away from the Active Recipient, who may either stand, sit or lie down comfortably, as they choose. The Initiator then begins to notice and then to follow his impulses towards the Active Recipient. It is crucially important that these are your impulses, Initiator, *in this moment*. Do not pre-plan your actions, and if possible don't censor them either. Some examples of gestures may be: to be in eye contact, to move closer, to take the hands of the Active Recipient, to give him/her a cuddle, to place your head in their lap, to give them a kiss, to caress them sensually, etc. Do this slowly and consciously, listening for the feedback of the Active Recipient, and responding appropriately.

- Active Recipient, you have a vocabulary of four important words: 1. 'yes' 2. 'no' 3. 'maybe' and 4. 'please'. You may choose from these four words when you respond to what the Initiator is doing. Respond to each of the Initiator's actions with one of the four words. If you like what the Initiator is doing, say 'yes'. If you don't like it, say 'no'. If you're not sure, say 'maybe', and if you're really enjoying or loving it, say 'please'.

- Initiator, you can't get this wrong – if you receive a 'no' from your partner, that's fine. You aren't trying to avoid getting the response of 'no'. The fact that your partner is taking care of their own boundaries, in fact, gives you more freedom to take risks, knowing that if they don't like it, they'll tell you. The aim is neither to necessarily fulfil all your unrequited desires, nor to necessarily please your partner. This is an opportunity to be responsive to your own feelings and impulses towards your partner, here and now, and to simultaneously respond and relate to them. This allows you to experience the mysterious 'third being', the relationship between the two of you. If you are feeling horny and cheeky and your partner is clearly feeling sensitive and sad, look for a gesture that will express your horny cheekiness and yet take your partner's sensitivity into account.

- Also if your partner says 'no', stop what you are doing and take a metaphorical, and perhaps physical step back and notice what happens inside you in response to your partner's 'no'. This is a very important and valuable opportunity for you to see the 'no' as a 'no' to this particular action at this particular moment, rather than as a global 'no' to you. It is not a rejection of you, or even of your behaviour as a whole, simply information and a request that the Active Recipient is not enjoying whatever is happening between you at this moment, for whatever reason. By the way, this is not a 'no' to this particular action for all time. Five minutes later you may feel inspired to do the same thing again, and this time you may receive a 'yes'.

- If your partner says 'yes', that means they are enjoying what is going on. You may continue with what you are doing, or change it. The choice is yours.

- If your partner says 'maybe', you can regard this feedback as meaning 'I'm not sure yet. Give me a little more time to decide.' In order that 'maybe' does not become an abdication of choice along the lines of 'I don't mind' or 'You choose', it is important, Initiator, that you *continue with what you are doing*, without progressing on to something else or retreating from this gesture, *until the Active Recipient has made a choice* between 'yes', 'no' or 'please'.

- If your partner responds with 'please', this means that they are really enjoying what is happening. Again, there's no need to continue with what you're doing, but you may like to!

- If your partner forgets to give you feedback – maybe they have got lost in pleasure – then simply and gently say 'hello', to remind them.

- When this turn is over, share another namaste, then swap roles without talking.

- When both partners have completed their turns, take some time to share, both of you, what you experienced in both roles. What did you discover about yourselves from relating in this way? What were your 'edges' or most challenging moments? What have you learned?

- If you like, you can proceed to have another turn each, integrating your previous discoveries. These second turns should be equal in time to each other, but may be longer or shorter than the first round of turns. Afterwards, again take a few minutes to share your experiences.

- Complete with a namaste.

One of my workshop participants, having enjoyed this exercise with her partner, introduced it to her two young children as an alternative to bedtime stories. Both children loved it, and in fact asked for it on many occasions. She discovered that one child preferred to be scratched, tickled and teased, whereas the other preferred to be cuddled and stroked. It has brought them closer as a family.

Roger and I have found this simple exercise surprisingly powerful. At times when we have had an argument and words have proved fruitless in restoring love and harmony between us, the 'yes, no, maybe, please' exercise has invariably succeeded in bringing us out of our minds, and into a direct bodily relationship in the moment. This has allowed us to reconnect with ourselves and each other in an intimate way, and has opened the space for constructive dialogue, if this is still needed.

Once you have practised the exercise on its own on at least one occasion, you may like to include it in lovemaking if you are in a sexual relationship. As you make love, take turns in being the Initiator and Active Recipient, and communicating as described before. Although it may seem a little contrived at first, this exercise imparts an essential principle, that of staying present in each moment and remaining in communication. After a while, the formal structure may no longer be necessary, and you can engage in lovemaking and life with the four words 'yes, no, maybe, please' in your awareness, as well as the principle of following your bodily impulses in a relationship with another person.

Yin-yang meditation: asking for what you want

The yin-yang meditation is an opportunity to embrace and explore our desires in the here and now. It is a place to let go of limitations to pleasure and go for what you really want, even if that is entirely different from what you thought you wanted. This meditation also offers a chance to recognise and discern between fantasies in the mind and longings from the body, when explored with your love partner.

I describe the yin-yang meditation in a sexual context. It can, however, also be enjoyed with a platonic or same-sex friend or friends. In this case you may choose to have a foot massage, or to have your hair stroked. You may also use it as a way of deciding what activities to engage in during your time together, such as a walk in the park or going out for a meal. You can be creative, letting the playful child within you have a say.

This is a very powerful meditation, one that may not at all times be entirely comfortable. This is congruent: you are exploring the possibility of extending your comfort zone, both as the active partner and as the supportive/receptive one, and you may feel the stretch. The meditation is best repeated at least three times, but preferably seven, during consecutive Tantric dates. In this way you can take some of the pressure off yourself: it isn't your one and only opportunity to really go for what you want; rather, it is a space in which to notice, and to become conscious of, your true longings in each moment, and for these discoveries to inform your sexual relating and your life.

The Technique

Decide how long each turn will be and how many turns you will have. This meditation can take anything between one and four hours. Ideally, if you can free up the time, have two turns at each role each, with the first 'round' of turns lasting half an hour per turn, and the second round lasting an hour per turn. With time to share afterwards, this will take three and a half to four hours. Decide who will be 'yin' and who 'yang' to start with.

- Share a namaste.

Yin

- Yin, your role is to be as fully present for yang as you are able to be, to support them in exploring their desires. You have an opportunity to really let go of your mind and become a devotee of yang. In this way you will be able to experience some of yang's world, to be initiated.

- You may be asked to do things or engage in pursuits that you would not normally choose to participate in. For example, you may be asked to stroke your beloved gently all over without that leading to sexual intercourse. Or you may be asked to take the lead in sex. If you are willing, even if not keen, go ahead and enter as fully into the experience as you are able to. Check in with yourself now and then to stay connected with yourself by closing your eyes, placing a hand on your heart and sex, and breathing into these places. It is important that you don't do anything that would be harmful to you. If you are unable to fulfil a request that yang asks of you, see if you can stay open to what you are able to offer them. Do not in any way mock or denigrate what yang asks you: always treat them and yourself with respect.

- Being yin can sometimes evoke perceptions of passivity or powerlessness. In fact, however, taking on the role of yin is entirely different. You are choosing to be receptive and welcoming of yang's impulses, for a reason and purpose of conscious exploration that ultimately supports you both. Take note if these feelings arise, breathe into them and remind yourself that you can choose to say 'no' if you need to. Some people find it an immense relief to be yin, a relief and a pleasure. Being yin gives you the opportunity to let go of striving and directing, and to sit back and respond with your love and sexuality.

Yang

- Yang, your role is to explore your desires in each moment. Ask yin for what you would like, for example 'I'd love you to give me a sensual massage,' or 'What I'd really like is for us to cuddle up, and for you to sing to me,' or 'I'd love to show you how much I adore you by covering you all over with kisses.' Your request, yang, may change at any given moment. See if you can allow your body, your heart, your aliveness in the moment to direct your choices, rather than any preconceptions of what you may have imagined, an hour ago, would bring you most enjoyment. In this way you will have an opportunity to find your natural pleasure impulses, and also to notice what, in you, gets in the way. You will have a chance to see what really nourishes and fulfils you, and what does not. You will be able

> to see what happens when you really ask for what you want, and stay in relationship, in communication, in contact with your partner.
>
> - After the allocated time for a turn is complete, share a namaste and swap round. When you have both had a turn at each role, you can either complete with a namaste and then take some time to share your experiences or, if you have decided on a second round, share a namaste and continue. At the end, take some time to share your experiences.

I loved being yin. It was really exciting. I loved being surprised by Pete's requests. At one point he blindfolded me and kissed and caressed me. I became unusually capable of receiving, receiving pleasure, and receiving Pete's masculinity.

Being yang was a nightmare for me. I tried to pack everything into my time, and managed to not really enjoy any of it. My mind was already planning my next exciting exploit, and it felt as if neither of us were anywhere. At one point I noticed Pete yawning, and I thought to myself: 'He's bored.' Of course, I then assumed that he was bored with me, and the whole thing plummeted even further. Afterwards, through tears, I recognised that I had received a big teaching. Actually, when it was my turn, I had been all over the place, and not really enjoying myself in the here and now. I saw that when I'm not present with me, Pete doesn't like it either. When I'm in myself, as I was when I was blindfolded, he really loves giving to me!

JANE, 50, REGISTERED NURSE

Love partners as well as friends can extend their range of possibility by exploring the yin-yang meditation outside of a sexual context. In this case, you can take turns in choosing how to do things. You can do this whenever you and your partner have free time together, or even while engaging in household activities such as cooking and cleaning.

Uncovering pleasure-limiting belief systems

Perhaps there have been times when you received the contact that you wanted, or were engaged in a pleasurable activity, but somehow you couldn't fully let it in. How does that happen? What do we do to limit our capacity to receive pleasure, and why?

Below is an exercise for couples that can help you bring to light some of these limitations, and in becoming aware of them to be in a position to choose whether or not to invest more energy in them.

The Technique

Take it in turns to give and receive the contact, cuddling, attention, touch and pleasure you would like. About thirty minutes to an hour each is ideal. You might like to be stroked delicately, massaged firmly, cuddled and kissed, erotically pleasured.

- Begin with a namaste.

- Ask for the touch/contact you would like, focusing on what is most pleasurable for you.

- As you are receiving, notice any thoughts or beliefs, emotions or body sensations that arise that impede your flow of in-the-moment enjoyment. These may take the form of:

    o Restrictive belief systems.

    o Feelings that are held back.

    o Tension (contraction) in your body.

- Breathe deeply, and welcome the thought/feeling/sensation fully. Notice how it affects your capacity to be completely present in the moment, and to enjoy pleasure.

- Share out loud the thought/feeling/sensation with your partner.

- Supporting partner, you simply witness what is being said. Continue to offer touch/contact/pleasure.

- It may be helpful for your supporting partner to write down your untransformed, pleasure-limiting beliefs. These can include:

    o I don't deserve it.

    o It's wrong to want pleasure.

    o Sexual pleasure is bad and dirty.

    o I'm afraid it won't last.

    o If I really let myself go, I might lose control.

    o Someone might see/hear/know.

    o Pleasure isn't spiritual.

    o I mustn't need anyone or anything.

    o It's so good I might cry. I mustn't be emotional.

    o I bet I look stupid.

    o I'll regret this later.

    o I should be giving, not receiving.

- As you notice and become more conscious of how you limit pleasure, you will less easily be trapped in this belief system in future.

- Return your attention to the touch and pleasure.

- Complete with a namaste.

- Take some time to share what has arisen. You may like to consider where the belief originated. Also ask yourself, 'Is there a possibility that this (belief) may not be the absolute truth?' or 'Can I open to a different, more life-affirming possibility?'

Having practised this exercise at least once, you can also begin to notice any anti-pleasure thoughts or beliefs that occur while you are making love. Common pleasure-limiting thought patterns in lovemaking can include trying to have an orgasm (for women) or trying not to ejaculate (for men), as well as wondering whether you're being a good enough lover.

By observing and becoming aware of the 'background noise' that limits your openness to pleasure, you may begin to take these beliefs less seriously, and to choose to return more quickly and easily to the enjoyment of life, in your body, here and now.

FROM PLEASURE TO BLISS

Once we have the capacity to open to pleasure here and now, we can take this a step further, and allow the pleasure to expand into bliss. Tantric touch, a very simple meditation, offers a potential insight into this experience. The keys here are being fully present in our body in each moment, combined with deep relaxation.

Tantric touch

When receiving a caress, Oh Princess, enter into it as everlasting life.

SHIVA SUTRA

A traditional and delightful Tantric meditation, the caressing meditation, or Tantric touch, is described below. You will need a partner, who need not be your beloved. This meditation is about purely receiving and purely giving Tantric touch. It is about letting go of the mind and sinking into our essence. As such, it is not primarily focused on the relationship between giver and receiver, but rather on each person allowing themselves to become as fully present in each moment as possible.

The Technique

A good length of time for this meditation is twenty minutes each way; an hour in total, including time for sharing. Other requirements are a warm room, a soft feather (ostrich or peacock are excellent), and some soft, meditative, wordless music.

- Decide who will caress first, and who will be caressed.

- Begin with a namaste.

- Receiver, tell your partner if there is anywhere where you would like them not to touch you. Then remove as much clothing as you feel comfortable with. This type of caressing is only really palpable on bare skin.

- If you are receiving for twenty minutes or longer, you may receive the caressing on both sides of your body. Start by lying on your front, so that you receive the touch on your back. If you have less time, choose one side to receive on, front or back.

- Giver, take the feather. Take a few moments to become comfortable and relaxed, sitting by the side of your partner, who is lying down. You are about to become like an extension of the feather, with all your awareness in the point of contact between the feather and your partner's body. When you are ready, begin to stroke your partner with the feather, starting at an extremity like a hand or foot, and continuing to cover all areas of exposed skin (except anywhere they have requested that you do not touch). Do this in one long, very light, very slow, continuous motion, hardly bending the tendrils of the feather as you do so. Treat each millimetre of available skin with equal reverence. Also include your partner's hair.

- After five minutes, continue caressing your partner with the same quality of very light, slow, conscious, continuous touch, this time with your fingertips. Use just one hand, and again treat each millimetre of skin with equal reverence. Remain relaxed and comfortable as you do this.

- After another five minutes, invite your partner to turn over, and repeat the feather and fingertip caressing for five minutes each on their front. If they are naked, include their breasts (for women!), yoni or vajra, but do not specifically focus on these areas. Let them be of the same importance as the rest of your partner's body.

- Receiver, there is nothing that you need to do, except to breathe in a full and relaxed way; any time that your mind wanders, bring it back to the simple sensation of the caress on your body.

- If you have more than twenty minutes, you can add one or two extra stages, with the same quality of slowness, softness, consciousness and continuousness. You may blow on your partner's body with either 'hot breath' (the type that you would use to steam up a pair of glasses before polishing them), or 'cold breath' (like silent whistling). Let your breath sweep over and caress your partner's body. Do not try to excite them or be clever. The breath (or caress) will enliven them, while the slow, continuous, gentle movement allows them to relax deeply into

> the experience. Other types of caress are with your hair, or with fur, or with your breasts or tongue.
>
> - When you have completed the caressing, allow the receiver to lie in silence, feeling their skin and the sensations in their body. Keep your attention with them, so that when they open their eyes, you are there to welcome them.
>
> - Complete with a namaste, then swap round.
>
> - After the second partner's turn is complete, share another namaste and take some time to talk about your experiences.

Touching in this way has several effects. One of these is to allow you to either fully give or fully receive touch. This can be a very relaxing and meditative experience for the giver as well as the receiver. It is not uncommon for the giver to almost feel the caress themselves. For the receiver, it can be a huge relief not to have to do anything or get anywhere, to just be.

The combination of very light, slow, continuous, conscious touch brings the attention of the receiver to their skin. It is as if their energy body expands to meet the touch. Because you are so relaxed, expansion is easy. Energetic expansion can be experienced as a sense of well-being, of joy, happiness or contentment. Although it is very fine, this type of touch can be intensely enlivening and pleasurable, in a whole-body sort of way. It is common for people who have received this sort or caressing to report that they could still feel the feather once it had been removed from their body, or that they couldn't locate the feather – it was almost as if it was everywhere at once!

The meditation awakens sensitivity. After you have practised it twice on its own, you can make love afterwards from this place of heightened sensitivity and awareness. I encourage you to continue to relax deeply, focus on whole-body pleasure, breathe fully and deeply and enjoy each pleasurable sensation at each moment.

CHAPTER TWELVE

SHAKTI MYSTERIES

In many traditional cultures, girls at the age of puberty used to and still do receive teachings and initiation rituals into the mysteries of female sexuality. In the West, however, the vital importance of sexuality as the ground of our being, as well as the integral role of marital and sexual union and fulfilment in the creation of a harmonious society, has been sadly lost and neglected. Tantra offers us the possibility of reclaiming the sacredness of what it means to be a sexual woman, whatever our age, and how to relate from this place inside us to our beloveds and to the world.

We can only find our identity as woman with and through women. When we can celebrate our own feminine sexuality without needing a man to affirm it, we are free. You may like to consider your answers to the following questions:

- How would I describe my relationship with myself as a woman?

- How do I relate to other women? What is good, healthy and life-affirming in my contact with other women? What is not?
- Where have my attitudes towards women come from?
- Which of my decisions about women come from my upbringing or past associations?
- What are my deeper wishes, hopes and longings in relation to other women, and towards myself as a woman?

As you start to unravel your attitudes towards yourself as a woman and other women, more space will appear for you to choose, from your heart and deeper wisdom, which of these really serve you in life. Tantra offers you a way to choose something new.

One way in which we can typically block our potential for learning and growing together as women, for finding what connects us, is by means of competition.

FROM COMPETITION TO EMPOWERMENT

When we see other women as our competitors and compare ourselves either favourably or unfavourably to them, we create a separation between ourselves and other women. When we can honestly recognise our own strengths and weaknesses, and celebrate our special gifts, then we can create a world of true empowerment and rich variety. The 'Shah!' exercise described below, combined with the theme of namaste, can dramatically transform some of our projections and comparisons into treasures.

The 'Shah!' exercise

You can do this exercise alone, with a pen and paper, or with like-minded female friends. The exercise itself is fundamentally the same:

in a group of women you have real-life people to engage with as 'mirrors'; on your own you have your imagination.

> ### *The Technique*
>
> This exercise can take anything from ten to forty minutes. It helps if you can be in a place where you feel comfortable about making some noise. I describe the exercise first as if you are practising it alone, and later say some words about doing it with others.
>
> - When doing the 'Shah!' exercise alone, imagine a woman with whom you compare yourself or feel in competition.
>
> - Visualise that woman standing in front of you, perhaps on a cushion, two to three paces away, and notice how you feel in yourself and towards her.
>
> - Greet this imaginary person with a namaste, acknowledging that she has something to show you about yourself.
>
> - Ask yourself about your hopes and longings, your intentions, relation to other women and this woman in particular. For example, you may wish to be truly free from the constraints of comparison, to feel your own worth and appreciate hers.
>
> - Take a deep breath and, when you are ready, as you exhale, swiftly and purposefully extend your right arm and leg in front of you, as you shout the sound 'Shah!', letting the sound come from your diaphragm, your third chakra. Imagine projecting your identity outwards, clearly, proudly and strongly, as if to say, 'This is me!' Make the extension of your arm and leg a fast and definite movement, like a flick-knife opening, and in that sharp way, communicate clearly with the gesture your presence and worth. Let the sound be similarly loud and definite, like

the cries emitted in martial arts, or as if a friend of yours was a long way away, just about to disappear out of sight, and you wanted to catch their attention.

- When the sound comes from your diaphragm, you can make it loud without straining your voice. It has a depth and resonance to it. Explore and experiment with breathing down into your diaphragm, and letting the sound come from there. You can pull in the muscles around your solar plexus sharply as you exhale, as if you have been punched and winded. Open your throat and let out a sound.

- Close your eyes and take some deep breaths, noticing any feelings or sensations in your body at this moment.

- Also become aware if you were able to extend your arm and leg and shout 'Shah!' while keeping your balance. If you lost your balance, did you topple forwards or backwards? What does this tell you about your habitual ways of asserting yourself?

- If you toppled forwards, this is equivalent to an energetic habit of losing your centre and becoming overly absorbed in another person, so that you forget who you are, your own worth and needs.

- If you toppled backwards, then part of you is projecting your energy outwards, and part of you is pulling away. In life you may experience this habit as one of giving mixed messages. You try to be clear, but can't really hold your ground in doing so. Perhaps you hate conflict. You say: 'This is me!' and then try to hide.

- Now imagine this woman once more in front of you. Notice how you perceive her. Has anything changed?

- Repeat the process once again, extending your right arm and leg and making the sound 'Shah!' from your solar plexus. Again close your eyes afterwards and notice any feelings or sensations in your body, and sensing your perceptions and feelings in relation to the woman you chose.

- Repeat the whole process twice more, this time extending your left arm and left leg in front of you as you shout 'Shah!'

- Again notice your own bodily sensations and feelings, and those towards your imaginary partner, sensing what has changed in you and your perception of her.

- Take some time to write down your experiences.

- Complete with a namaste, honouring once more this woman as a mirror for you.

Advanced 'Shah' exercise

Having practised 'Shah!' alone, you can experiment with a real person.

The Technique

- Before you begin, share with each other in what way you compare yourself with her, and what your intention is for this practice.

- Both do the exercise simultaneously, counting to three and shouting 'Shah!' together.

- After each round, share with each other what has changed in you.

Shakti mysteries

The first time I did the 'Shah!' exercise, at a women's workshop, I knew immediately the woman who was making me feel inferior, and I made a beeline towards her. She was a tall and beautiful strawberry blonde (who I'm sure had naturally hairless legs!) and she was confident, sensual and sexy, and intelligent and creative to boot. I knew that if there was a competition between the two of us for a man, she'd win. Worse still, she knew it too. Well, I can't explain exactly what happened during the course of the exercise. I remember a great sense of exhilaration and power as we 'Shah-ed' at each other. I felt that we were matched in our passion, and that, like lion cubs, we were sparring and playing with each other. I noticed my attitude towards her softening, and I saw a real person beneath the rather two-dimensional, statuesque perception I had held of her. I sensed that she felt and saw the real me, too. What I certainly know is that at the end I felt a warmth towards her, and although I still admired her incredible combination of looks and gifts, I felt that I had touched her humanness too, and that made all the difference. I could enjoy being inspired by her, without diminishing myself in the process.

This exercise mobilises and releases tensions in the solar plexus, the central manifestation on a physical level of the third chakra (*see page 106*). The third chakra is concerned with our sense of identity and individuality. It is as if we are empowering the phrase '*This* is who I am! I am proud to be me!' As with most Tantric exercises and meditations, be prepared for feelings to arise! I did this exercise when I needed to fire an office staff member who I liked a lot, but who wasn't right for the job. I was very nervous about asking her to leave, and as I continued with the 'Shah!' exercise I came more deeply in touch with the origins of my fear of asserting myself. Paradoxically, though, being more in touch with my vulnerability helped me to do what I needed to do in a humane way.

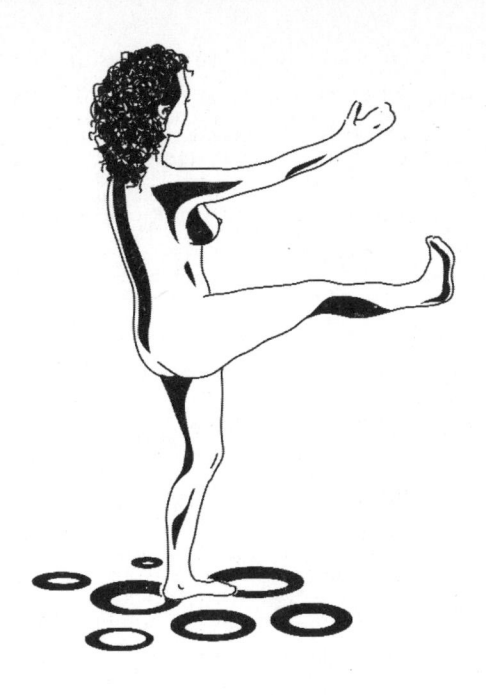

THE SHAH! EXERCISE

TANTRA FOR WOMEN

Having laid some foundations for our identity, self-image, confidence and connectedness as sexual women, we may now go on to celebrate our full, feminine, sexual-loving potential.

OUR BEAUTIFUL BREASTS

Our breasts are the erotic manifestation of our hearts. As women, we are positively charged, that is, ready to interact with the world from our hearts (*see pages 133–4*). It is therefore congruent that our breasts extend from our bodies. They are the place from which we are able to feed and nurture a baby. There is much that we can do to look after, celebrate and explore the erotic, loving and energetic potential of our breasts.

Breast massage

Massage and bodywork in general are becoming more mainstream as a means to enhance health, well-being and relaxation. I was lucky enough to train with a very holistic school of massage, where we learned about the importance of treating the body and person as a whole, and massaging in long, sensual strokes to bring integration and pleasure to the recipient. Then, after nine months of training, came the time for our exams. Suddenly the brief changed and we were learning techniques to massage just one body part at a time, along with intricate manoeuvres with towels to maintain modesty. The examination board, it appeared, believed in professionalism, not holism.

Even in the most holistic of therapeutic and professional massage schools, breasts and genitals are excluded from the treatment, and for good reason. There are enough difficulties for bodywork professionals to face around boundaries and clients' subconscious processes without introducing erogenous zones into the picture. However, this does exacerbate the general split between receiving touch for relaxation and rejuvenation, which must exclude erogenous zones, and touch as a turn-on and prelude to sex, which often focuses almost entirely on these areas. A healing breast massage can do wonders to restore this balance, recognising the potential for sexual pleasure that our breasts can afford us, celebrating this, and yet orientating itself towards health, well-being, care, relaxation and healing.

Breast massage is something you can do for yourself, or it can be a delightful gift to receive from a lover. In the latter case, breast massage can be included as part of a whole-body massage.

IMPORTANT NOTE: IF YOU ARE PREGNANT, DO ONLY GENTLE BREAST CARESSING, WITH NO DEEP MASSAGE OR LYMPHATIC DRAINAGE, AND DO NOT INCLUDE BREAST ROTATION (*see page 186*). Pregnancy is a time when your breasts are meant to swell and retain fluid, and it is best not to interfere with the new hormonal balance that is being established. Also avoid these techniques if you have breast cancer, and consult your doctor first if you have any other type of breast disease.

The Technique

The breast massage takes about twenty minutes, and requires a warm room, some massage oil and some gentle music if you like. You (or your lover) must have short fingernails. I describe the massage as if you are massaging your own breasts.

- Use only a minimal amount of oil, so that your skin isn't too slippery. A few drops is generally just enough to allow your fingers to slide comfortably over your skin without causing friction burns. Warm the oil between your hands, and lightly apply it to your breasts by circling them with your palms.

- Start with one breast first. Caress or gently squeeze your nipple. Enjoy the pleasurable sensations that this evokes.

- Then, just at the edge of your nipples, apply firm but sensitive pressure to a point on your breast next to the nipple. Gently circle the tissue underneath, with your fingers still in contact with the same bit of skin. In other words, you aren't sliding over the skin, but rather massaging the underlying areas. Do this for about ten seconds, or longer if you experience tenderness. Keep going, perhaps more gently, until you feel the tenderness lessen or disperse in some way.

- Next, move your fingers a couple of centimetres radially out from your nipple, and repeat this procedure. Continue in this way, moving radially out from the nipple at two-centimetre intervals until you have gone just beyond the outer edge of your breast.

- Return to just outside the edge of your nipple, at a point just next to where you started, and repeat the circling, moving in a radial direction as before. Continue in this way until you have covered the whole of your breast.

- Now move to the other breast and repeat the same process.

- With both hands and both breasts together, stroke the underside of your breasts from in between them out to your armpits. This enhances lymphatic drainage.

- Rub your hands together until they are warm and energised. Place your palms on your breasts and, holding them lightly, circle them upwards and outwards. This forms part of the Taoist 'deer exercise' for stoking your sexual fire. The Taoists suggest circling in this way for at least thirty-six rotations.

- Slowly and consciously remove your hands from your breasts, then take a couple of minutes just to notice how your breasts feel.

A lovely gift to yourself, and part of a yummy self-care programme, is to massage your breasts each week. Your breasts will look forward to that time, and thank you for it!

Breast meditation

Massaging your breasts will prepare and sensitise them, and allow them to maximally enter into this traditional Tantric meditation, the breast meditation. This meditation develops and matures within you. Ideally do it ten times within a time frame of a month at the most, or better still, every day for ten days.

Feel the fine qualities of creativity permeating your breasts and assuming delicate configurations.

SHIVA SUTRA

The Technique

Sit comfortably, somewhere quiet where you will not be disturbed, for twenty minutes. Ideally, do this meditation naked, or with your breasts unclothed. It is fine also to do it fully clothed.

- Close your eyes and allow your body to relax.
- As you breathe, bring your attention to your breasts.
- As the sutra says, simply become aware of any sensations, images or senses that you receive from your breasts, and in the space around them.
- There is nothing in particular for you to 'get'. Just be here and witness!

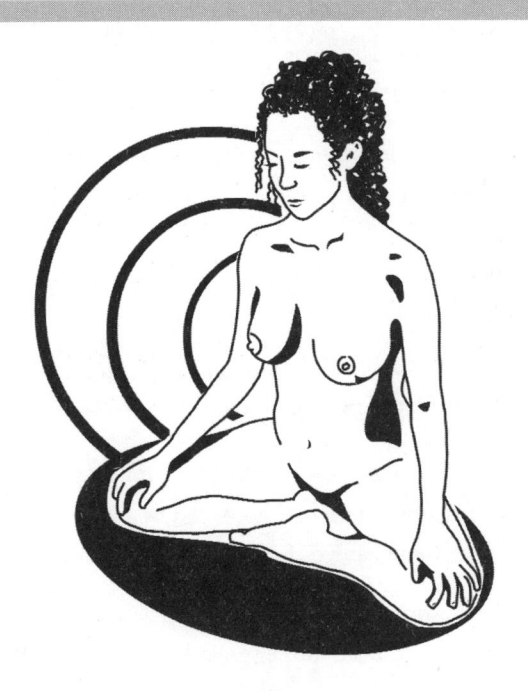

BREAST MEDITATION

YONI WISDOM

The word yoni means 'sacred place'. This translation conjures up very different connotations from 'vagina', 'pussy' or 'cunt'. It is for us as women to recognise, honour and celebrate the sacredness of this place in us.

Admiring yoni

I recommend repeating this meditation which you do alone, three times, to notice how your attitudes and feelings towards yoni evolve with awareness and time.

The Technique

The meditation takes about twenty minutes. You will need a medium-sized hand-held mirror, some sexual lubricant, and a pen and paper.

- Undress and spend a few moments cupping yoni, breathing down into her, and noticing any sensations, feelings or messages that she is communicating to you.

- Position the mirror so that you can see yoni. Look at her from the outside. As you breathe, gaze at yoni with soft focus, receptive gaze, allowing yourself to be curious, and welcoming whatever thoughts or feelings bubble up.

- When you are ready, part yoni's outer lips and gaze at her inner regions, as before with soft focus, allowing yourself to be curious and noticing whatever thoughts and feelings arise.

- Anoint yoni with some lubricant, and gently stroke and explore her. If she becomes aroused and engorged, that's great. If not,

> that's great too. Just be with her, allowing your childlike curiosity and playfulness to guide you.
>
> - Bid farewell to yoni for now, and return to cupping her, closing your eyes.
>
> - Gently remove your hands, open your eyes, and take a few minutes to write down your experiences.

The first time I really looked at my genitals, I had the startling realisation of what was actually there. Being brought up on the notion that boys have penises, outside, and girls have vaginas, inside, actually ignores the fact that women have external genitalia – our vulva or yoni. In some cultures they literally cut out women's genitals; in ours, we do so symbolically. I knew there was a hole, but looking presented me with a whole new picture. Wow! So much more than a hole!

Having trained as a fertility counsellor, I was used to looking at my cervix through a speculum, a plastic tube that opens inside the vagina, and a mirror. For years I had looked yet not seen – not until I attended a women's sexuality course.

I was surprised to see such delicacy and intricacy, the different colours and shapes. The fuzzy splurge of pubic hair, the oval-shaped outer lips and the differing shapes of the two inner lips. Opening my inner lips revealed another aspect – my clitoral bud and the butterfly shape of my inner lips.

Did you know that the clitoral bud is just the tip of the clitoris? When I touch this place I can feel the length and breadth of my whole clitoris. We have erectile tissue spreading from our buds to our anuses and the width of our lips.

Shakti mysteries

> *Yoni at rest and yoni aroused are two different beings. I love looking at her and exploring all her folds and curves, getting to know what to touch, how and where turns me on. Inside is my G zone, which is especially sensitive and orgasmic.*
>
> *Nowadays, as a psychosexual therapist I encourage clients to look in detail at their genitals, to befriend a unique and intimate part of themselves. Often people feel that others, doctors or lovers, have seen in detail what they have not. Beginning to see and feel the changes we go through during sexual arousal helps to recapture the wondrousness of our bodies and our sexuality. Instead of shame, they feel pride. I love my 'passion flower'.*
>
> CABBY, 47, PSYCHOSEXUAL THERAPIST AND FERTILITY COUNSELLOR

Yoni gazing

This traditional Tantric meditation is one to be shared between love partners. It may not sound like much, but it can transport both Shakti (meaning 'goddess', the woman) and Shiva (meaning 'god', the man) to a different, peaceful and yet mystically alive realm. The aim of the meditation, however, is simply to be with the thoughts, feelings and body sensations as you (Shiva) gaze at yoni, and as Shakti receives Shiva's gaze.

After you have experienced the yoni gazing meditation at least once, you may like to repeat the meditation and make love afterwards. Whether or not you follow the meditation with lovemaking, ideally repeat this meditation three times.

The Technique

The meditation takes twenty minutes. You need to be warm and comfortable.

- Undress, both of you, and share a namaste.

- Shiva, offer a namaste to yoni.

- Shiva, indicate to Shakti a position of your choice in which you would like to gaze at yoni. Shakti, make sure that you are comfortable.

- Shiva, find a comfortable position from where you can gaze at yoni. Simply gaze in silence, as you breathe, and notice whatever thoughts, feelings or body sensations arise in you. Do not follow trains of thought or fantasy, just 'name' what you are thinking or feeling, such as 'arousal' or 'embarrassment' or 'wonder', and continue to bring your attention back to yoni. Allow yourself to simply be here, now, with yoni.

- Shakti, allow yourself to be with how it is for you that Shiva is gazing at yoni. Again, gently return your attention to the here and now, your body and breath, whenever it wanders. Name the thoughts and feelings that pass through your mind. Allow yourself to sink gently into simply being Shakti.

- After about twenty minutes, Shiva offer a namaste again to yoni, and then Shakti and Shiva share a namaste.

- Do not talk about your experiences for at least half an hour afterwards. Just 'be' with the experience.

You can only gaze like that if you feel honoured, experience a reverence for Shakti, and for yoni. It is the complete opposite of pornography, which is like a 'yoni on a stick', rather than a real, sexual woman. For yoni gazing, you have to be aware of the whole person. When I am calm, quiet and attentive, the yoni I normally see becomes just the tip of a sexual iceberg; as I become silent and gaze, I find myself entering into the whole sexual being of my Shakti.

DENNIS, 45, DOCTOR

Before we began, I wondered if I'd feel like a sex object. I wasn't sure if I liked the idea of even my husband peering at me in that way. But as soon as we shared a namaste, and he greeted my yoni with a namaste, I thought, 'No – this is different.' In fact, it was so different that I felt quite tearful for a while. It was one of those 'aha!' moments. I knew that this was how it was meant to be. There was a timeless quality to the meditation. I felt sexy, regal, young, old and peaceful.

RENEE, 36, BUSINESS DEVELOPMENT TRAINER

Tantra is about seeing the sacred, the universal, in the everyday world. Yoni gazing is one of the most direct routes to experiencing this, as the mystery in yoni is so readily apparent if we allow our minds to quieten down enough. If you, as a woman, have ever shown yoni to your young son or daughter and told them that they came out of there, you will probably see the amazement on their face. It is amazing, the mystery of birth. In the cavernous depths of yoni, this sacred place, you may glimpse the dark expanse of the Universe.

CHAPTER THIRTEEN

SHIVA WISDOM

This chapter was written with Dr Roger Lichy

As part of my Deep Diving Tantra training, the men and women spend time separately on several occasions. This is described in the programme, and in general it is the part of the training that the men least look forward to. Some feel very cautious, not liking the idea of 'male bonding', and are concerned, particularly in a Tantric context, in case it involves any homosexual activity.

In actual fact I'm not that surprised that the men are wary. Few heterosexual men have a model for or an understanding of the potential in spending time with men, without any homosexual undertones, and with an openness to being seen for who they really are. My hope is that this chapter will offer you a glimpse of what that potential may be for you, as well as an appreciation of some of the principles involved in men's sexual healing, and in Tantric Shiva wisdom. Although it may appear (in particular when I speak about issues concerning homophobia) that I am predominantly addressing heterosexual men, it is simply that homosexual men may not face the same issues when opening up to other men. In fact, however, all of the exercises are equally applicable, whatever your sexual orientation. They will help you find a deeper, fuller, more expansive and sacred sense of masculinity.

MEN'S SEXUAL HEALING

Roger says, 'If, as men, we try to get our identity from women, it will never work. We become dependent on women and impoverished as men.' When a man knows that he is dependent on a woman in a way that goes beyond the natural interdependency that we reach in intimate relationships; when a man knows, underneath whatever his personality portrays, that he is relying on women for his sense of worth as a man, his manliness, his raison d'être, then deep down he will resent her. This is not an ideal starting point from which to engage in Tantric meditations of Union, and yet this state of dependence may be a natural consequence of his history. Let us now look back in time.

When a baby boy is born, his mother is all-important. For him, she is the Universe, the source of life. It is she, in most cases, who predominantly feeds and nurtures him. After nine months within her body, an energetic umbilical cord continues to serve mother and baby for some time post-partum. This accounts for many mothers' acute sensitivity to their baby's needs.

At a certain point, however, early in childhood, boys realise that they are different from their mothers. Realising that they are not the same as the central figure in their universe can be a huge shock. It is not possible, therefore, for a boy child to find his male identity in his mother. In order to discover who he is, and what it means to be a boy who will one day become a man, he first needs to energetically put some distance between himself and his mother, and then to find his father.

In today's culture, this is no mean feat. The mother may be

anything from ideal to 'good enough' to critical to overbearing, to in any other way neglectful or simply not good enough. The quality of early mothering that a boy receives, and the willingness of his mother to release him to his father, and to let her son know that she will still be there when he wants her, will all influence the ease with which this step is taken.

Then there's the father. It seems to me that a lot of boys are left in a vacuum, needing to separate from their mothers, but unable to make adequate contact with their fathers. If the father works long hours, is overbearing, critical and frightening to his son, or is in any other way emotionally unavailable to meet his son's needs, that boy will encounter difficulties in establishing his identity. If a man didn't get his identity needs met as a child, the good news is that he has an opportunity to do so as an adult.

OUR SEXUAL ORIGINS

Below are some questions for you to reflect upon, relating to your development as a sexual male. Bear in mind that these questions may evoke some very deep material. If you are in any way emotionally or mentally challenged at this time, or if you know or suspect the presence of trauma in your childhood, save the exploration of these questions for when you are in the presence of a professional therapist or counsellor.

You may like to write down your answers as they arise in a journal or on a piece of paper. Substitute 'mother figure' for mother, or 'father figure' for father, if either parent was absent. Consider too the impact of this absence.

- When you were a young boy, between the ages of three and seven, how was your relationship with your mother?

- When you were a young boy, between the ages of three and seven, how was your relationship with your father?

- How available were your parents for physical and emotional contact?

- Did your mother support or hinder your relationship with your father? In what ways?

- How did your mother and father respond to your penis, and your emerging interest in it?

- As you reached puberty, how did you experience the presence and support of your mother and father?

- What messages, advice, or information did your parents give you about sexuality and maleness, in words, deeds or in what wasn't spoken about or enacted?

- What has been the impact of these experiences on your adult life as a sexual man?

- In an ideal scenario, what would you have needed to be different? What difference would that have made in your life?

In Tantra workshops, we explore some of these themes and offer opportunities for you to 'reparent' yourself, gaining a new, wholesome, supportive inner sense of masculinity. Adrian's account below shows some of the benefits he received from doing this.

> *I was on a week's Tantra holiday course abroad. Early in the week it seemed as though a few of the women were feeling antagonistic towards a couple of the men, and we separated out into men's and women's groups to address what was coming up. I was annoyed at first. My idea of Tantra was about being intimate with women, not men, and I was very resistant to the 'father stuff'. I thought I'd been there, done that, anyway.*
>
> *But then something changed. I was talking to my 'father' and found that there were tears streaming down my face. He had been a rough man, an angry man, and I had been afraid*

to express any tender feelings towards him. As the man who was pretending to be my father listened to what I was saying, I really had a sense of my father, who had died three years earlier, in front of me. And when he talked back to me, as my father, it was so real. It was just what I wanted to hear. I asked him for a hug, a manly hug, and it was so nice, so safe and strong. I felt his power protecting me, and I felt proud to have him as my dad.

And something else, when all of the men had gone through this experience, and the women had done whatever they were doing, we reunited and exchanged gifts, and all the animosity had gone. What was particularly fascinating to me was that it mattered less what women thought of me, now that I could feel my father here with me.

ADRIAN, 45, ARCHITECT

MEN AND TOUCH

When I was a psychology undergraduate, I once saw a picture in an American social psychology textbook. It depicted outline figures of men and women, shaded in areas where they most commonly received touch from members of their own and the other sex; the figures were of heterosexual men and women, in both social and intimate settings. The more darkly shaded areas represented more contact. Without going into all the details, the 'men touching men' picture was noticeable by the absence of any shading, except for on the hands (darkly shaded) and on the back (presumably from patting – it was very lightly shaded). The 'women touching women' drawing, by contrast, showed a far more varied shading over the whole of most of women's bodies. I imagine this is not terribly surprising to you, yet it made an impression on me. Why is it that women have licence to enjoy caring, non-sexual physical contact from each other, whereas men do not? And anyway, why should men want to touch other men, when, hopefully, they can receive touch from women?

I leave you to find your own answers to the first question, and focus on the second, to begin with by giving you some questions to consider. You may contemplate the answers to these questions, write them down or share them with a friend.

- How would I describe my relationship with myself as a man?

- How do I relate to other men?

- What are my fears about receiving touch from other men?

- What could be the potential benefits for me?

- What is my 'comfort zone' around men and touch? What is comfortable for me, what is not and what am I not sure about?

- Which of these decisions come from my head, my ideas, and which come from my body, from a source of deeper wisdom?

As I have said before, contrary to many ideas about Tantra, the point of it all is not simply to push away all your previous barriers and inhibitions. The value is in discerning which of your attitudes and approaches to life stem from your history or conditioning, and which are fundamentally true for you. This is an almost impossible question to consider in your mind; only doing, sensing and feeling your way, in the appropriate setting, will ultimately bring you these answers. In doing so, you will become freer to be who you truly are.

> *As we talked through our ideas, fears and the potential benefits of receiving touch in the form of massage from men, I practised what I had learned in Tantra, to 'sit with my resistance'. This meant noticing that I have some negative ideas about it, specifically some fears, and yet not acting on those fears. I could also recognise an opportunity that I had not had in this way before, to try out a new way of being with men. Eventually, reluctantly, I took the plunge. It was the trust that we had already built up, as a group of men,*

> *and my knowledge that the others shared similar fears and intentions, that allowed me to do it. I felt safe with them. At first I still felt awkward. All sorts of thoughts popped into my head. I kept reminding myself to come back to my body. About halfway through I relaxed, and then it felt fine. In fact, more than fine. I'd call it 'wholesome'. It reminded me a bit of being in a men-only Turkish bath in Turkey, being massaged and scrubbed by men. It felt quite normal, this masculine environment where men just hung out together as men.*
>
> Jeremy, 33, IT Consultant

The difference between homosexual activity and male contact is primarily one of intent. The intent of the former is to become sexually aroused, perhaps to the point of climax. In the second, your intention may be for contact and presence, healing/transforming your relationship with men, discovering a nourishing way to receive touch from men, sinking deeper into your experience of masculinity or just to enjoy simple, non-sexual pleasure.

While receiving touch, it is possible that vajra may become erect. This does not necessarily signify sexual desire or attraction. In this context, this is highly unlikely. As you know, vajras become erect for all sorts of reasons, like when you are feeling alive in your body. All-over body pleasure will often include some erection in vajra. The question is not what vajra does, but what your mind does with that. If you are really worried about getting an erection, you will not be present enough to experience the touch! If you do get an erection, your mind can make all sorts of stories out of it, and make it mean all sorts of different things. This is where a simple body sensation becomes sexualised, made to mean something more than it actually is.

Roger says, 'For centuries, sexually explicit touch has been commodified. More recently, in the Western world, non-sexual massage has become available in professional settings. The social value of non-sexual, nourishing touch appears, however, still to be undervalued. Touch is a fundamentally natural way to give and receive loving contact. Young children who grow up with parents who are at home with touch instinctively know whether to go to Mummy or Daddy for physical interaction, cuddles or play.'

Coming out of the cave: men's massage

This is an exercise that you can explore with two male friends.

The Technique

You will need some massage oil and some massage towels. The massage will take one and a half hours, comprising thirty minutes per turn.

- Begin with a three-way namaste.

- Decide who will go first. Number one, take five minutes to talk about your fears, your hopes and your intentions for receiving touch from other men.

- Number one, remove as much clothing as you would like to. If you would like to remove all your clothes, first check with the other two Shivas that they are also comfortable with this. They are unlikely to be able to offer you loving touch if they themselves are uncomfortable.

- Let them know where you would and would not like to be touched, in what way, and by whom. You can, for example, be very specific and ask one man to massage your feet and legs, while the other massages your back and chest. You can massage with oil, or choose firm, reassuring touch (without oil), lighter touch or more nurturing contact like a hug.

- Supporters, make sure that you are in your truth, and that you are also happy to give what is being asked of you. If you are not, say so, and let the receiver know what you would be happy to give. Touch with the quality of presence with which you yourself would like to be touched.

- Supporters, begin gently and consciously. Be comfortable in your own body, and spend a couple of minutes breathing in time with the receiver, to harmonise with him, before making physical contact. Remain aware of each other.

- At any time, receiver, you can choose to be touched differently. You can give feedback, asking for more or less pressure, and so on. Once you have chosen, simply relax, breathe and notice how you feel. Notice any thoughts, feelings or sensations that arise in you. Keep bringing your attention back to the physical contact, your anchor in the here and now.

- Become aware of the quality of male touch. How does it differ from female touch? What do you miss about female touch? What does male touch bring you that female touch does not?

- After twenty minutes, find a place of completion. Supporters, bring your hands to rest for a minute or two before disengaging slowly and consciously, keeping your attention with the receiver until they open their eyes.

- Number one, make eye contact with your two supporters, receiving and thanking them with your gaze. Notice how you feel in this moment of eye contact, in this recognition of the tactile contact you have shared.

- Take five minutes to talk about your experiences in receiving touch. Supporters, take five minutes between you to share how it was to give touch.

- Complete with a namaste.

- Move on to Shivas two and three.

> *There was a sense of loving firmness and strength that put me back in touch with myself.*
>
> ROB, 57, RESTAURANT MANAGER

TANTRA FOR MEN

What does it take to satisfy a woman in sex? My suggestion is, forget about satisfying her; look to fulfil her by finding fulfilment in yourself. She will be fulfilled when she really feels your presence, your openness and vulnerability, honesty and power, when you make love. It is about bringing your heart into your vajra, and the best way to practise this is through the male breath (*see page 135*), and this is what will also fulfil you, as you make love as an expression of your true masculinity.

Vajra meditation

What will also enhance and elevate the experience for both of you is having a keen awareness of vajra, both in terms of his physicality and in terms of his essential, archetypal qualities. Here is a meditation to support you in developing these different levels of awareness in vajra. You can either do the short form of the meditation, or take it further as described below.

> ### The Technique
>
> You will need about fifteen to twenty-five minutes at a time when you will not be disturbed.
>
> Sit comfortably with your back erect, preferably cross-legged on a cushion, or on a seat where you are not leaning on anything. Close your eyes and take some deep breaths. Gradually allow your awareness to settle in vajra.

- Begin with a namaste to yourself, your Shiva essence.
- As your awareness rests in vajra, begin to 'feel into', get a feeling sense from the inside, of the different parts of vajra. Feel into your balls, the root of vajra, his shaft and head.
- Notice the subtle differences in the qualities of sensation in these areas.
- Keep bringing your attention back to the sensations in vajra. Let yourself deepen into them, as if you are becoming vajra. This is the essence of being a man, being Shiva, being vajra.

Advancing the meditation

- Now imagine that your entire body has become vajra, so that your head is vajra's head, your body is the shaft of vajra, your legs are the balls and root of vajra. Welcome impressions, sensations or feelings that arise in you as you do this.
- Let yourself now become the universal male principle, that penetrating force that desires and can make love with everything on the planet. Imagine yourself as this universal vajra making love with the earth, the trees, the flowers, rivers, lakes and seas. Let yourself make love with caves.
- As you focus on your head, your crown, imagine making love with the sky, black holes and spiral nebulae, the universal yonis in the cosmos.
- Gradually, from wherever you are in your consciousness, let yourself return to the here and now, the man that you are, with a sense too of still being vajra. Notice how you feel about yourself, about life, about making love, about vajra.
- Complete with a namaste, with gratitude to whatever aspects of your being, of your Shiva essence that have become available to you today.

Roger says of his experiences: 'After doing this meditation, I can remember a release of my anxiety about whether it was OK to be a man with strong sexual feelings. For the first time in my life, I felt a huge "YES" inside my genitals, filling me with joy, filling me with energy. For the first time in my life, I felt enormously proud of being a man.'

Another man who did this meditation, Rob, was delighted to have permission to recognise his pan-sexual nature, and felt for the first time able to distinguish between the Shiva principle that *does* want and is able to make love with everything that moves, as well as having the desire and capacity for a committed long-term, one-to-one sexual, loving and spiritual relationship. Paradoxically, by recognising this universal Shiva principle in himself, he felt more relaxed and expansive, and more ready and willing to commit himself more deeply in his relationship with his partner, without having to act it out.

THE ENERGETIC BASIS OF MASCULINITY

It can be very difficult these days for a man to know how to be. He's supposed to be gentle, tender and heartful; to cook, wash up and look after the children. That's on top of working, bringing in money and after all that being a sex god in bed. On the one hand it appears that women want men to be more like women, yet on the other hand they want men to be 'real men'. Is this an impossibly mixed up cocktail, or is there a secret formula that can bring all these ingredients together? And anyway, what do men want?

Energetically, a man is positively charged in his genitals and receptive in his heart (*see page 130*). It is therefore not advantageous to try to 'be in your heart' in the way it is for a woman, but rather, to be in your balls: to be in your true power and authority, and to bring your heart into it.

So, if a woman wants you to listen, listen to her, and stay rooted with your awareness in your base. That way she won't knock you over with her emotionality and you'll be able to hear her without having to defend yourself, even if you don't like what she's saying. You will feel better, more manly, more detached, and yet freer to really reach out.

Vajra root meditation

Here is a meditation that can provide you with a varied range of experiences, all of them positive. Examples of these benefits are given after the description of the technique below.

The Technique

The meditation takes between fifteen and twenty-five minutes, and requires just a quiet place to sit, with your back erect. It can be helpful, before you begin, to touch with your fingers the area of the root of vajra, where he enters into your body. If you press firmly into your perineum point, the soft place just beyond vajra root, you can also touch, feel and sense the root of vajra inside your body.

- Begin with a namaste to yourself.

- Take some deep breaths, and bring your awareness down to the root of vajra, where vajra enters your body.

- Sense the place inside your body where vajra's root begins. Place your attention in this place. As you breathe, let your awareness arrive more and more deeply here.

- Notice any feelings or sensations that arise. If you feel any tension or discomfort, gently encourage it to melt, to let go. Keep breathing and noticing whatever you feel, softening into it.

- After a while, you may notice a gentle tingling or vibration in your pelvic floor, your vajra root. Allow this vibration, tingling or warmth to spread into the whole of your pelvis.

- This is your main positive pole as a man. It is your connection with your life-force energy and the life-force energy of the Universe. Celebrate it!

- Finally, imagine a circle of energy between this positive pole, your base chakra and your opposite positive pole, your crown. Notice what this is like, connecting in your body the place where you connect to life-force, and the place where you connect with essence, Spirit, Great Mystery.

- Just rest here for a few minutes, with your awareness lightly resting in both poles and the connection between them.

- When you are ready, return to a sense of your physical body in the room. Complete with a namaste, honouring yourself and your energetic potential.

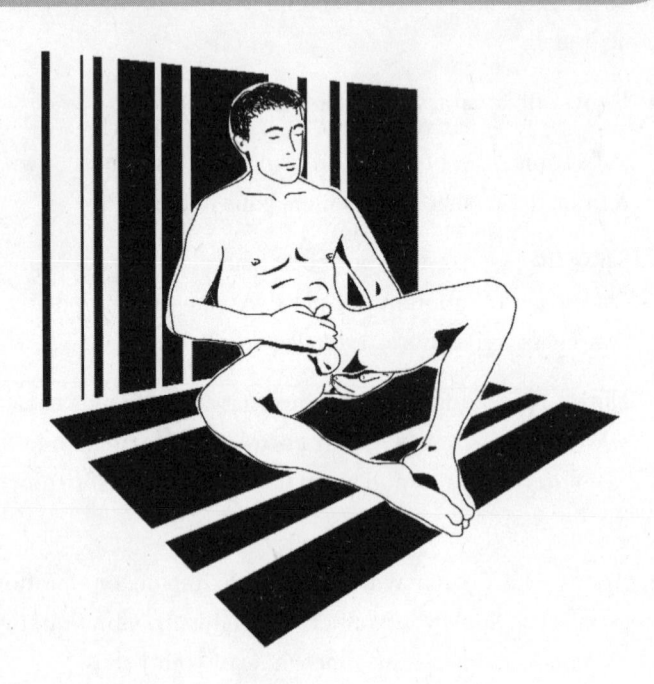

VAJRA ROOT MEDITATION

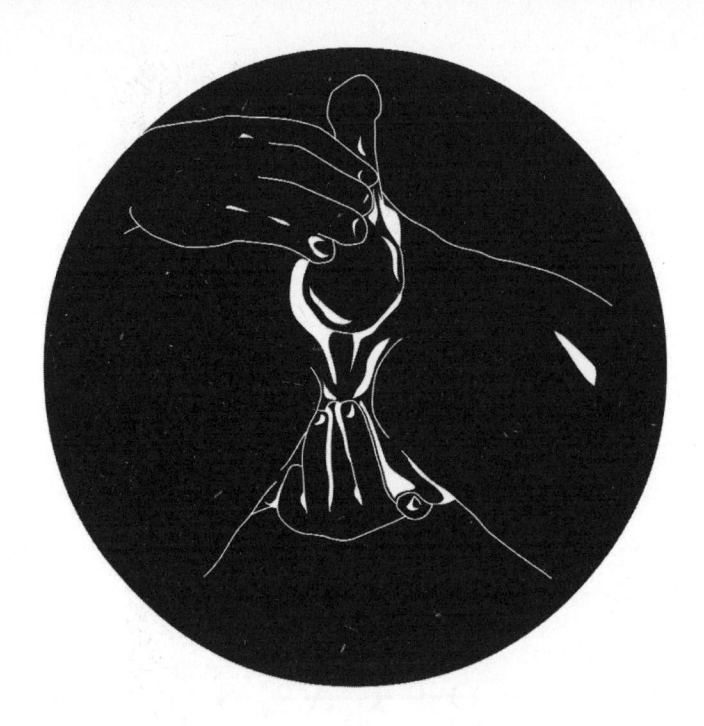

LOCATING THE VAJRA ROOT

As mentioned men who have practised this meditation have had a varied range of experiences, invariably positive. Tom found that in connecting with his base chakra he could think more clearly and be more creative and spontaneous, and that it gave him more energy. Jeremy says that discovering his vajra root in this way is like finding his 'man's heart'. For Dennis, it was the soul of vajra that he clearly sensed.

Having explored the questions, exercises and meditations in this chapter, it is likely that you will be on firmer, more self-aware and rewarding ground to continue with some of the more advanced Tantric meditations offered in the following two chapters.

CHAPTER FOURTEEN

OUR SACRED SEXUAL ORGANS

This chapter is devoted to our sexual organs, our relationship with them and their integration with the rest of our body and being.

HEALING OUR GENITALS

Did you masturbate as a child or teenager? What happens for you as I ask that question? Do you imagine a critical parent about to scold or shame you? Do you feel ashamed, or comfortable and proud?

It is entirely natural to explore and touch and feel and enjoy our genitals, both as young children and later, in a different way, as adolescents. There are rare cases of young children who masturbate continually, usually as the result of another emotional issue, but these are in the minority. In general, young children touch and pleasure themselves, and then get on with playing with their cars, construction games, computer games or dolls, or with painting or dressing up. For them, there's no big difference, no big issue.

At workshops, when people talk about their early experiences of masturbation I hear stories of young children being smacked, told that they will go blind, or being punished or humiliated. I hear stories of adolescent secrecy, of masturbation in socks or towels or silently under the covers, with the fear of further retribution never far away. What do you imagine it would have been like if these people had just been allowed to get on with it? Our genitals are ours, after all. This is our own sexuality we're talking about; it's here to be explored!

As we reach adulthood, it's often more of the same. The word masturbation is laden with shame and value judgements. Insults such as 'you jerk' or 'you wanker' reinforce the perception that people who masturbate are sad nerds, slightly deranged or otherwise undesirable. For this reason, I prefer to refer to masturbation as self-pleasuring. Self-pleasuring is one of a family of positive expressions of self. This family includes self-awareness, self-acceptance, self-respect, self-expression, self-love, self-care and self-pleasuring. Self-pleasuring can be a celebration of our selves, of our capacity to feel and give ourselves pleasure.

That is not to say that all masturbation is healthy. When we have been shamed for giving ourselves pleasure, we may repeat a way of treating ourselves that mirrors our early conditioning. If masturbation is shameful, and yet feels good, feels really good, then we'd better do it in secret. And hope that nobody finds out. And feel bad about it afterwards. We may wiggle or stroke our bits in an urgent attempt at release, while not really feeling much pleasure in the process at all. Many of us touch ourselves in a way in which we would hate anyone else to touch us. Masturbating in this way is more akin to self-sabotage than to self-love.

So it's up to us now to set things straight, to transform masturbation into self-pleasuring, to allow self-pleasuring to become an indication, a celebration of self-love, self-care and self-expression.

Self-love and self-pleasuring

The subjects of loving ourselves (Chapter 10), and reclaiming the beauty and sacredness of yoni and vajra (Chapters 12 and 13) have already been covered. This is the backdrop for transforming masturbation into self-pleasuring. You are now ready to create a self-pleasuring ritual, to celebrate yourself and your sexual pleasure.

Remember that in entering into a self-pleasuring ritual with yourself, you are challenging a huge taboo in Western culture. Don't be surprised if you feel discouraged, embarrassed, numb, distracted, bored, lonely, frustrated or impatient at times. This is normal. As you embrace how you feel, breathe and keep coming back to the here and now, it will change. Remember the principle of 'what you resist persists', and how to heal shame. Remember that transformation happens through really seeing, knowing, feeling and recognising the extent of our past pain and past conditioning, and then choosing something new, something pleasurable, in the here and now. Having really engaged with the preceding exercises of self-love and vajra and yoni honouring will make this next step more fluid, easy, natural and joyful.

I would recommend, to begin with, not using a vibrator. For now experiment with a softer, less intense sort of pleasure. If you want to pleasure inside your yoni and can't reach comfortably with your fingers, use a dildo or a vibrator without the vibration!

As the most important theme here is to love yourself as you are, being loving and compassionate towards yourself is more important than experiencing sexual pleasure. It may be, for example, that as you breathe between your sex and your heart, you feel the longing for a sexual partner, or a type of sexual intimacy that you have been missing. That grief is real and valid. It is part of your journey of recognising your true longings, and reclaiming your integrated sexuality. Let yourself feel sad. Cry if you need to. Hold or cuddle yourself, curl up under the duvet. Whatever your impulses are, follow them. When this wave of sadness, or whatever you are feeling, has passed, return to pleasuring yourself. Be sensitive to your needs at this moment, and what it is that truly brings you pleasure.

Try also to avoid the self-sabotaging pattern of having unrealistic expectations. If you have felt numb and non-sexual for a long time, don't expect some candles and sexy underwear to turn you back on. A realistic expectation in this situation would be to love yourself regardless of how sexy you feel, and to look for when and where you feel little glimmerings of pleasure and notice what stops them from growing and igniting.

Finally, I recommend for this ritual that you refrain from using fantasies that are about you being somewhere else, in a different context, with someone else or other people. Explore letting your passion come from your body, rather than from your mind. If you have fantasies, let them be real-life images of you pleasuring you, of your inner lover and beloved. Let your mind and imagination enhance and engage with what is really here now.

The Technique

You will need at least two hours in total for the ritual, in a time and place where you will not be disturbed. Why not make an evening of it? Items that may enhance your ritual are: a special outfit, some flowers, massage oil, a good sexual lubricant (*see* Resources, *page 250*), a cloth or sarong and a blindfold. You may also like to prepare some music, which will play for the whole time, with a range of fun, sensual, upbeat and gentle tunes.

- Imagine that you are preparing for a very special date, a date with you. Prepare the room so that it is inviting and sensual, comfortable and beautiful. You may like to buy yourself some fresh flowers, set out beautiful cloths or sheets. When you are ready to begin, light incense and candles.

- Shower or bathe and put on your special outfit. Look at yourself in the mirror, and let yourself know how beautiful you look. If you like, take a photograph of yourself, or ask someone else to do so, to remind you.

- As you enter your sacred space, sit in silence for a few minutes, allowing your mind to settle. Reconnect with your intention for engaging in this ritual. Invite your inner lover to be here with you, that part of you that can delight in giving and receiving pleasure with yourself. Welcome and greet your inner lover with a namaste.

- If you like, you can blindfold yourself. This helps you to focus your attention inwards.

- Stand or remain sitting, and begin to move or dance. Find the enjoyment in your body that movement brings. There is no right or wrong way to dance; let your bodily impulses guide you.

- In your own time, do a striptease for yourself. Again, don't think about how you look; instead just let yourself turn yourself on.

- When you are naked, continue to move as you touch, feel and caress your skin. Notice how your body feels to the touch of your hands, and how you feel beneath your own caress. You are at once the lover and the beloved.

- When you're ready, you can sit or lie down and, if you like, anoint yourself with oil. Whether or not you use oil, take time to greet and welcome each little part of your anatomy, from your toes to your bottom to your face and hair. Leave vajra or yoni till last.

- If you are a woman, take some time to massage and caress your breasts.

- Cup vajra or yoni with your hands, breathe into him or her, and anoint vajra or yoni with lubricant. Do this in a loving and sensitive way, in the way that you would like a lover to do.

- With one hand caressing or cupping vajra or yoni, place the other hand over your heart chakra area, in the centre of your chest. Breathe between sex and heart, heart and sex, as in inner flute breathing (*see page 143*). Notice how integrated these two places feel in you, and however you experience yourself, gently allow this connection to deepen, with your breath, hands and contact.

- As you caress vajra or yoni, be present in your touch. Let your inner lover touch you in the ways that bring you most pleasure, from a place of love. Feel each movement, and delight in the sensations. If you wish to take yourself to orgasm, you can do so any time. In the meantime, really enjoy the ride!

- Experiment with pleasuring vajra or yoni with one hand, and touching another part of your body with the other hand, feeling the connection between the two. Try gently touching your third eye.

- Also, when you feel a build-up of arousal in your pelvis, explore allowing it to spread through your body by stroking it down your legs and up your torso, and breathing fully and deeply.

- Experiment with keeping your arousal levels moderate. If 10 is orgasm, and 0 is no arousal at all, play with somewhere between 5 and 7. In this way, your sexual pleasure has more chance to gently trickle into the whole of you, rather than getting stuck purely in your pelvis. Perhaps bring your hand away from vajra or yoni at times, and breathe, move or lie still, feeling your body, being with yourself.

- You might like to explore combined pleasuring (*see page 216*).

- Remember your playful inner child – this ritual is for you to enjoy the process, rather than to achieve any particular goal! Have fun, be light, play.

- Orgasms are up to you. You may end with an orgasm, end without an orgasm, end after several orgasms. Do whatever brings you most pleasure, aliveness, ease, relaxation and joy. The ideas in your mind of what is pleasurable, and the knowledge and feelings in your body, may be different. Trust your body.

- To complete, sit or lie with one hand cupping vajra or yoni, and the other hand on your heart. Breathe once more between these places in a relaxed way.

- End with a namaste to yourself and your inner lover, thanking yourself for taking you on this journey of self-pleasuring, with love.

This is a ritual that you can repeat on many occasions. It is likely that each one will be different. The magic is in being in the moment.

> *Now that I am used to self-pleasuring as a self-honouring activity, two things have changed. Taking responsibility for my own orgasms makes for a much better balance with my partner, since he does not feel such an obligation to produce one. Also I enjoy taking my time much more, enjoying pleasure just for its own sake, and am far more prepared to experiment. Something that Roger said, too – try just noticing and enjoying the beauty – opened up something very important and special for me.*
>
> EVELYN, 65, RETIRED PUBLISHER

SEXUAL PLEASURE

Sexual pleasure can occur as part of sexual intercourse, and you can also devote time to specifically giving, and at other times receiving, loving sexual pleasure through touch, massage and pleasuring. At any time, should a pleasure-limiting belief or emotion arise, you can refer back to the 'uncovering pleasure-limiting belief' exercise (*see page 171*). In the Deep Diving Tantra workshop programme, we practise giving and receiving genital touch purely for healing, before focusing on pleasure. One of the fundamental aspects of offering a healing genital massage is for the giver to be fully present for the receiver, letting their hands become extensions of their heart.

The hands are extensions of the heart massage

It makes all the difference in the world whether you give pleasure mechanically or as a means to the end, or whether you do so from a joyful connection with your own love and sexuality. When we offer pleasure from our true being, the experience has a quality of fun, curiosity and spontaneity. When you share loving touch, you may desire to please your beloved as an expression and celebration of your mutual love and sensual, sexual delight. This is entirely different from seeking to turn on your partner simply in order to prove yourself as a great lover. When the hands are clear vehicles of love that is both given freely and received graciously, then pleasuring already becomes a deeper, more spiritual experience.

Many of the exercises and meditations in this book have the potential to reconnect you and your beloved with your sexual-loving flow, and as such can help you find a conducive 'inner space' to give and receive pleasure. The male and female breath, for example, is fundamental. Chakra breathing meditation will help to bring you into alignment within yourself and together as a couple. Vajra or yoni gazing are a beautiful precursor to giving pleasure. In fact, anything that helps to bring you more fully into the present moment will bring you into love.

The Technique

- Begin with a namaste.

- As you make contact with the skin, body, vajra or yoni of your beloved, close your eyes and breathe.

- When giving pleasure, Shiva, as you inhale, let your heart be filled with the love you have for Shakti. As you exhale, let that love travel down into your vajra. As you inhale, breathe the potency of your sexuality into your heart (*see page 129*). Imagine that the sexual love circulating within you is spreading from your heart into your hands, so that your hands express both your love and your presence, your pleasure in giving pleasure.

- When giving pleasure, Shakti, feel down into yoni. Imagine the delicious sensations that you have known in yoni are rising up to your heart as you inhale. As you exhale, imagine that your love is flowing from your heart, down your arms, into your hands and into Shiva's body and vajra.

- Experiment with letting your hands touch and caress your partner's body and genitals from the impulses that arise in you, out of your own love and pleasure. Don't plan, or try to achieve anything, just let your hands and body, heart and sex guide you.

- Receiver, remember the principle of the 'yes, no, maybe, please' exercise (*see page 163*), and give your partner some verbal or non-verbal feedback now and then. For instance, you may moan or say 'mmm' if you're enjoying it, or 'a little softer please', or whatever you need to say to communicate your need for something to change.

- Be open to and curious about each moment, rather than trying to direct your partner. Be open to receiving and appreciating as fully as possible what comes.

- Complete with a namaste.

My wife of thirty years, Gill, and I had not made love for almost as long as I could remember. I had stopped even thinking of her as a sexual woman. She was more like a sister to me, or sometimes a little girl. In our couples' Tantra sessions, Leora spent some time guiding Gill into connection with her own body and truth, through a solar plexus meditation, and then by doing a sensual dance for herself. I must admit that I was quite shocked. I had never seen such an expression of womanly sexual desire on her face before.

On the next occasion that we met, Leora once again guided Gill into herself, and I could see the look on her face and something about her posture change again. Gill announced that she would like to give me pleasure. I didn't know whether to whoop with delight or to run out screaming. I almost couldn't handle this turn of events, but I went with it. For a long time now, I had felt immensely irritated when Gill touched me – I can't tell you why. But this time, it was fine. I didn't flinch or cringe or shoo her away. I let her stroke and massage me all over. I let her touch my vajra and pleasure me. It was so long since anyone aside from me had done that, that I had to hold myself back from taking over. She seemed strangely confident. When I opened my eyes for a moment to glance at her, she had that look about her again, that womanly look. I couldn't let her bring me to orgasm – that would have been too much – but I was flabbergasted enough as it was. I think that was the first time ever that Gill had pleasured me as a sensuous woman.

> *Before she had been trying to please me, but I knew that she wasn't really enjoying it, and my body couldn't stand that.*
>
> SHANTI OWEN, 56, TRAIN DRIVER

DEEPENING PLEASURE AND BECOMING MULTI-ORGASMIC

Having established an attitude and ground for giving and receiving pleasure, below are some ideas to play with. I would recommend that rather than being formulaic or trying to do it right, you let your intuitive impulses, your love and spontaneity, guide you, and use the following suggestions as a source of new ideas and inspiration. I describe pleasuring your beloved with your hands. You are welcome, however, to include and combine manual and oral pleasuring any time that you choose. If you do include oral pleasuring, I recommend using an 'edible', water-based lubricant, such as Eros waterformulation (*see* Resources, *page 250*) rather than silicone-based lubricants.

Shakti's delight

Shakti, receiving pleasure is a receptive, and yet not passive role. You are in charge of asking Shiva for what you would like and what you don't like, and generally communicating how you feel, in order to stay present in each moment. It is also up to you to breathe as freely as possible, and to move and make sounds that welcome and enhance your pleasure. Relax and enjoy the ride! Any time you notice yourself becoming tense or anxious, pause and share this with Shiva. Take a deep breath and exhale with a sigh. The more that you relax, the more the pleasure in yoni can spread into the whole of you.

Shiva, the first time you offer Shakti pleasure, refrain from making love afterwards, unless she absolutely wishes that to happen. Let her know that this pleasure is for her, and you are not expecting anything in return. Once she knows that pleasuring isn't necessarily a precursor to penetrative sex, Shakti may choose to bring the experience of pleasuring, the aliveness, delight and orgasmic feelings, into lovemaking. You will find that this enhances and deepens the lovemaking for both of you.

Rather than writing about 'orgasms', I focus on helping you to become more 'orgasmic' in pleasure, in lovemaking and in life. If you are hoping to discover your orgasmic potential and have not previously been able to have orgasms, then understandably, having an orgasm may be a goal of yours. Paradoxically, however, trying to have an orgasm is unlikely to get you one. In contrast, relaxing and focusing on fully receiving pleasure in the moment may open you up to this side of you. Be patient, and keep noticing when and how you tense up, contracting your vaginal and surrounding muscles, when you go into your head and begin thinking and analysing, etc. When you notice precisely how and when and why you start to resist the experience of pleasure, this awareness will open new doors of possibility for you. Being orgasmic is living in an ongoing flow of scintillating aliveness, feeling the pulsation of life in your veins.

The Technique

This exercise will take around one to two hours. You will need (if you choose) massage oil, lubricant, towels, and (Shiva) very short, smoothly filed fingernails!

- Begin with a namaste to Shakti.

- Shakti and Shiva, share your intentions for this time together.

- Start with an all-over body massage, commencing on her back, using long, sensual strokes. Give particular attention to her buttocks, loosening up the muscles here and around her sacrum, the triangular bony plate at the base of her spine. Then ask Shakti to turn over, and massage the front of her body, a little more delicately.

- Alternatively, start with some whole-body Tantric touch, as described on page 173.

- Spend plenty of time caressing Shakti's breasts. These are her positive pole, and are generally ready to receive touch and pleasure before yoni is. Caress the whole of her breasts first, before focusing on her nipples. Ask Shakti what brings her most pleasure.

- Offer a namaste to yoni. As you do this, have your intention in mind for offering this gift of pleasure to Shakti.

- Form a bridge between yoni and Shakti's heart.

- Shiva, cup yoni, while Shakti, you breathe down into yoni and bring your awareness into her.

- Shakti, you direct Shiva. You are in charge; Shiva is in loving devotion, while remaining in his integrity.

- Shiva, you can gently squeeze Shakti's outer lips together, massaging them. Your intent here is to elicit the most pleasure in Shakti, rather than specifically to heal yoni. Remain in dialogue with Shakti, as you explore together what, at each moment, she enjoys most.

- Be open, at any time during the massage, to entering the spirit of healing, should an issue that is ripe for healing spontaneously present itself. If a painful sensation, emotion or limiting belief arise, encourage Shakti to breathe into whatever she is feeling, staying fully present with her. Pause in the massage, staying in contact with Shakti and yoni while you do this. When the wave of healing is complete, return to 'stalking' the pleasure.

- Anoint yoni with lubricant. Use plenty of it. Caress yoni very gently – this will help to awaken sensitivity combined with relaxation here.

- Let Shakti guide you.

- As you caress the external area of Shakti's yoni, let yourself become fully present in the touch. Feel and enjoy the soft moistness of her 'passion flower'. Express the love and delight you have for her and her yoni.

- Sometimes pleasure yoni with both hands; at other times use one or both hands to caress Shakti's whole body, her belly and heart and breasts; her face and hair; her thighs and legs.

- Come into eye contact frequently, and breathe together.

- Ask Shakti, now and then, 'How is this for you?' or 'How would you like me to touch you here?' or 'Is there anything that you would like me to do differently?' It's a dance between you being fully present in your love, truth, sexiness and desire to love and give pleasure to Shakti, and yet remembering to communicate and be receptive to her wishes, and respectful of her needs and feelings.

- Before entering yoni with your finger, ask permission to enter. This asking permission can be very healing, and can develop a deep trust and respect between you both. Shakti, whenever you are ready, invite Shiva's finger inside yoni.

- Explore pleasuring Shakti's pearl, or clitoris, at the same time as stroking her goddess spot (usually behind the pubic bone on the front wall of yoni). This is called blended pleasuring. Generally, pearl offers a more direct, localised, sharper experience of arousal, whereas yoni and the goddess spot feel deeper, more diffuse, more intimate.

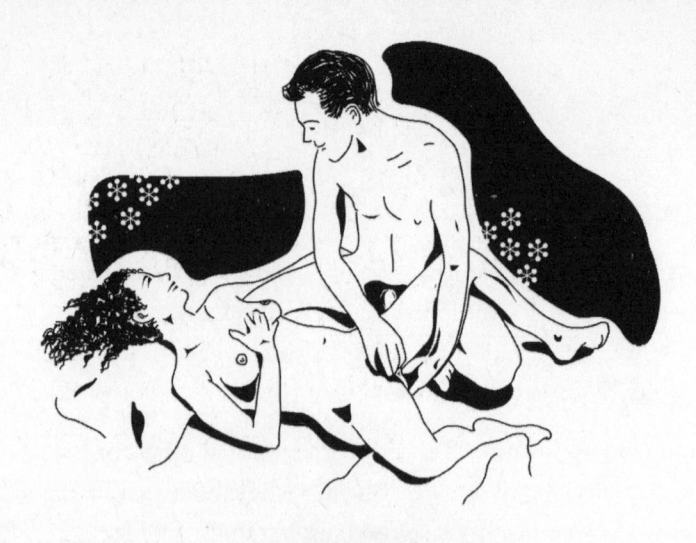

SHAKTI'S DELIGHT

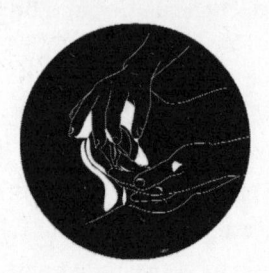

STROKE HER GODDESS SPOT AND PEARL

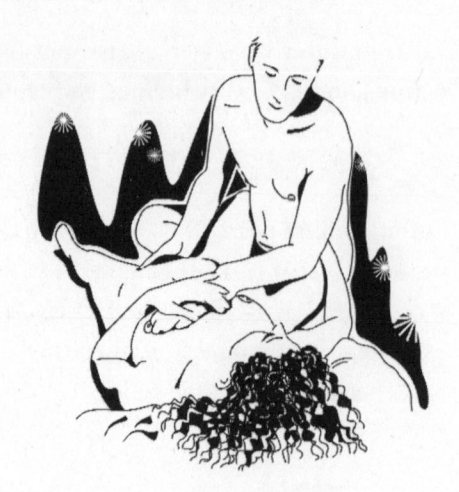

FORMING A BRIDGE BETWEEN SHAKTI'S YONI AND HEART

222 — TANTRA

- Shakti, imagine that you are allowing yoni to open wider and wider. Alternate sometimes, gently squeezing your love muscle as you inhale with fully relaxing and softening yoni as you inhale. This will help you remain aware and engaged with yoni and your breath, and may remind you to relax and let go!

- Remember, you are not trying to get somewhere or achieve something, aside from being fully present and opening to the pleasure that is here now.

- Guide Shiva with your words.

- Share your experiences with Shiva – this will help you both to be more present and alive.

- Be open to ripples of pleasure, involuntary vibrations both in yoni and in the whole of your body. Let go into these.

- Shiva, if Shakti has an orgasm, touch only very lightly, or refrain from pleasuring her pearl for a short while, and focus instead on her goddess spot. Shakti has the potential to continue to experience orgasms, so don't stop just because she's had one, unless this is what she chooses. Be open to more pleasure, whether that takes the form of specific 'orgasms' or not.

- Shakti, you are in charge, and you direct what Shiva does, and yet I encourage you to surrender to yourself. To let go and trust your body. To relax and open.

- Carry on for as long as you choose. When it is time to withdraw your finger from yoni, Shiva, do so slowly, consciously and lovingly.

- Cup yoni and Shakti's heart. Breathe together. Come into eye contact.

- Shakti, ask Shiva for the contact that you would like from him, perhaps a warm cuddle and kisses.
- Complete with a namaste.

Some women find that when pleasured in this way, they ejaculate. Yes, it's true. Women too can ejaculate. Female ejaculate is a clear fluid emitted from the urethra by some women while highly aroused and receiving protracted pleasuring of their goddess spots. It is generally emitted in spurts of liquid, varying in volume. This fluid has been shown to be different in make-up from urine, and is thought to originate from the spongy erectile tissue surrounding the urethra. It is this that you are pressing upon when you massage Shakti's goddess spot.

> *It was so wonderful just to receive, and to feel truly honoured. I was on cloud nine for the rest of the week!*
>
> DOMINIQUE, 42, TRANSLATOR

Shiva's delight

The first time you do this ritual, refrain from making love immediately afterwards in order to allow Shiva the chance to simply receive and be honoured, with nothing else required. If, in future, you do continue to make love after pleasuring, it is generally a good idea to pleasure Shakti first, then Shiva, and for Shiva not to ejaculate! Again though, see what works for you.

The Technique

Allow about one to two hours. For items you may need, refer to Shakti's delight (*see page 219*).

- Begin as for Shakti's delight, namely sharing a namaste, voicing your intentions, giving Shiva a delicious whole-body massage or touch, and then offering a namaste to vajra.

- Cup vajra and Shiva's heart, forming a bridge, and breathe together, coming into eye contact.

- Anoint vajra with oil of a silicone-based lubricant.

- Caress the whole of Shiva's perineum, inner thighs, vajra and belly with long, sweeping strokes.

- As you pleasure vajra, return frequently to strokes where one hand is pleasuring vajra, and the other is making contact with another part of Shiva's body, such as his belly, legs, chest/heart area, third eye or face. At these times, Shiva, let your awareness be in both places at once, forming a 'pleasure bridge'. Let your breath be full and relaxed, a vehicle for expanding pleasure.

- Joseph Kramer, a Californian pioneer in the area of erotic touch, says that the penis is the most touched organ of a man's body with the least creativity. He describes many ways to caress vajra that do not lead directly to ejaculation. These include:

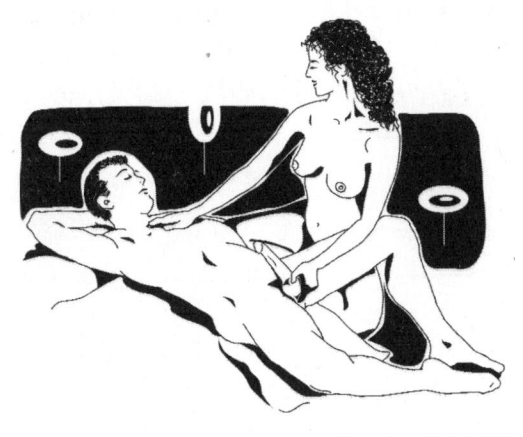

1. CUP VAJRA AND SHIVA'S HEART

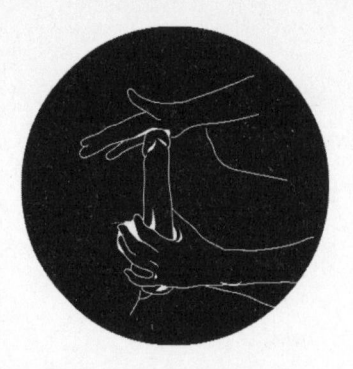

2. ANCHORING VAJRA AT BASE, FORM A 'RING' AROUND HIS SHAFT, GENTLY RUBBING HEAD WITH OTHER PALM

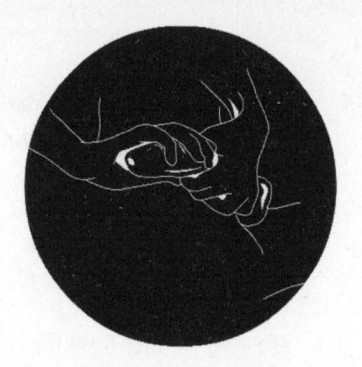

3. TWISTING LIGHTLY IN OPPOSITE DIRECTIONS, UP AND DOWN VAJRA SHAFT

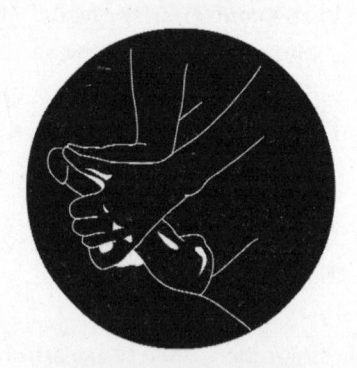

4. ALTERNATE THUMB CIRCLES AT RIDGE OF VAJRA HEAD, ESPECIALLY AROUND THE FRENULUM. FORESKIN PULLED BACK

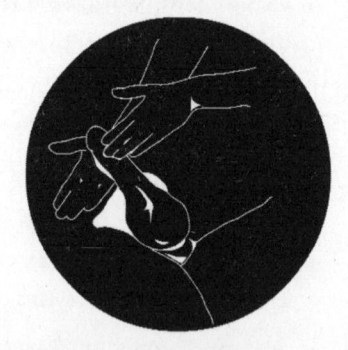

5. RUBBING VAJRA BENEATH BOTH HANDS UP AND DOWN SHAFT

- Shiva, remember to breathe in a full and relaxed way and to stay present in the moment. Remember also that you are in charge. If you're not enjoying yourself, don't blame it on Shakti – change something, either in how you are receiving the touch, or in how you direct Shakti.

- Shakti, also make sure that you are fully present. If at any time you notice that you are not, ask yourself what it is that you need, or need to do in order to return to the here and now. Don't be afraid to pause in the pleasuring to recentre yourself. If Shiva asks you to do something and you cannot, with integrity, agree, tell him. In this way, you continue to give pleasure to Shiva with genuine love and generosity.

- Every now and then, Shiva, you may like to pause and focus on spreading the energy around your body. You can ask Shakti to stroke up to your heart and third eye, and simultaneously breathe into these places.

- Experiment, Shiva, with relaxing into and containing the sexual energy, letting it suffuse your cells in the ways described above. In order to do this, I recommend keeping your level of arousal well below the point of no return. If you surf the edge of ejaculation, then tension can build up in your genitals, which is neither pleasant nor particularly healthy.

- I also do not recommend pressing the perineum to avoid ejaculation, as recommended by some. This again is not healthy, is quite mechanical, and does not come close to the art of relaxing into and fully enjoying pleasure. When you are able to sustain pleasure and let it also become love and bliss, you can enjoy the 'valley orgasm', which is more of a continuous rippling of pleasure throughout your body, or orgasmic experiences that are not genitally focused and do not necessarily include ejaculation. You may be inspired to read the accounts of some of these experiences later in this section.

- When the time comes to end, you can either complete with an ejaculatory orgasm, or simply relax into the experience and let the pleasure permeate your body.

- If Shiva ejaculates, you may also continue giving him pleasure with vajra soft or semi-erect. This can open up a whole new range of experience.

- When you are complete, Shakti offer a closing namaste to vajra, and find some way to be together, such as cuddling.

- Before you move on to other activities or sleep, close with a namaste.

> *My whole body became alive and sensitised, so that even the slightest touch of vajra would send ripples through the whole of my body. And the rest of me became super-charged too. A hand on my chest, a butterfly kiss on my cheek, all produced ecstatic bursts of joy in me. There was a stage when I wanted to ejaculate, but kept relaxing deeply and breathing through my inner flute. And then the sense of urgency for an orgasm went. It was a bit like running through a stitch and coming out again into second wind. It's as if I emerged into a 'pleasure zone'. This feeling stayed with me for hours, and in a more subtle way, days afterwards.*
>
> ROB, 57, RESTAURANT MANAGER

Tantra is about entering deeply into the sacredness of what's already here, and our sex organs are here, and sacred, whether or not we're 'doing Tantra'. It's just a matter of whether we choose to be open to that fact. Loving touch massage to vajra and yoni can heal, and be a sharing of pleasure and a gateway to whole-body bliss. Enjoy!

CHAPTER FIFTEEN

SACRED UNION: integrating sex, love, relationship and spirit

In truth, every body is the Universe.
MAHANIRVANA TANTRA

When you have established a grounding in bodily awareness, a compassionate attitude towards yourself and a sense of your energetic identity as a man or woman, when you have discovered and taken responsibility for your own pleasure in vajra or yoni and its overflowing into the whole of your body, when you are familiar with the approach of namaste, where you see your partner as a teacher, a mirror, and when, at least at moments, you can love them for who they really are and not just who you want them to be, when you can sense the Universe in your beloved's eyes and in yourself, then you have already tasted Union. Union is where you are in your essence. When you and another being are both in touch with your essence, and you meet from this place, this too is Union. It is where two personalities drop away and something greater, that is everywhere at all times, takes over. According to Ram Dass, a brilliant and amusing American spiritual teacher who spent many years with an enlightened master in India, it's like stepping into a hot tub of grace with another person.

ECSTASY

I want to know if you can be with joy, mine or your own, if you can dance with wildness and let the ecstasy fill you to the tips of your fingers and toes.

ORIAH MOUNTAIN DREAMER, *THE INVITATION*

Ecstasy is an expression of Union, of oneness. To be ecstatic does not just mean to be extremely happy; it means leaving your ordinary mind behind; it is about transcendence. It is about entering so fully into an experience of the moment that we enter the realm of timelessness. Our hearts and minds open and we become love.

The Greek origin of the word ecstasy is *ex stasis*, to move beyond stasis. In Latin, *ex stare* means to stand outside oneself. As Tantra teacher Margot Anand says, ecstasy is 'glimpsing the infinite'. In a sense, all Tantra is ultimately about ecstasy; it is about following our hearts and the truth of our bodies, and moving beyond the rigid limitations imposed by our minds.

Ecstasy is about entering so deeply into everyday phenomena that we touch what is Universal. We experience sacredness within the mundane.

> *I once lay in the grass, looking up at the sky, and became aware of being the ground. There was nothing between the sky and the earth – I was the earth. I experienced a total at-one-ness, which was blissful.*
>
> MIKE, 42, COMPUTER ANALYST

'Every moment is pregnant with ecstasy,' says Margot Anand. We do not have to go searching for it. We can allow it to take us, when we are open to it.

SEXUAL ECSTASY

Sexual ecstasy happens when the pleasure, joy and intimacy of sex expand to the degree that we experience a perceptual shift; we open to a greater experience of ourselves. Clarity and Bob had been together for two years. Previously Clarity had been in a marriage in which, for the last four years, her husband didn't want to have sex. She had become very serious, and quite passive. Until she met Bob, who was spontaneous and passionate.

They came to Tantra to find fun, pleasure, physical sensations and integration. They also hoped that Tantra would bring them even closer. Clarity had never been able to experience orgasm, but she had let go of looking for a solution some time ago, and this was not the reason that she came to Tantra. She was sceptical of the idea of 'chakras', but was willing to go along with the more 'esoteric' stuff because she so much enjoyed all the rest.

About halfway through the Deep Diving Tantra training, an ongoing series of workshops attended by the same group of people over seven months, Clarity and Bob were at home, making love. Quite spontaneously, Clarity had her first orgasm. Of this she says the following.

> *I was fully present in my body, and in the experience of pleasure, love and bliss. I was allowing my body to lead me, and all of a sudden there it was. Powerful, glorious, ecstatic!*
>
> *Before that moment I hadn't allowed my body to be so much in command. My mind is very strong, and I love my strong, imaginative, creative mind. I am highly educated, and through this, my mind has been nurtured to the exclusion of my physical, sensual body. But it interferes with*

> *intimate moments. It has a grip on me, and can transport me completely out of an experience. I had noticed feeling frightened just before this moment of 'leaving my body'. I'm sure that's because my mind is afraid of letting go of control. I'm used to being in control.*
>
> *In my marriage I was always controlling my feelings and what I said. Now I've decided to be more spontaneous, and I like it better, even though speaking my mind can be quite hair-raising sometimes. Our relationship has been tested many times, and yet each time it has become stronger. A lot of the time I'm tired because of hepatitis, which developed into fatigue, and I think that's because my mind had been driving my body. My body just conked out through self-neglect and pushing myself. Now, though, despite all that I feel happy – and at moments ecstatic even. Ecstasy for me is the pinnacle of letting go of my mind, whether that's in sex or in anything else.*
>
> CLARITY, 36, ARTS MANAGER

In letting go of her mind's control by trusting and relaxing into her bodily reality, Clarity was able, in sex and in life, to go beyond her previous limitations, to become ecstatic.

RELATIONSHIP YOGA

Romantic novels, women's magazines and films can lead us to believe that fulfilling, ecstatic relationships can appear on a plate, if only we are able to find, and keep, the right plate. This attitude predisposes us to feel like failures, to become resigned to a life of mediocrity, to decide that we chose wrongly and return to the marketplace in search of the elusive 'perfect partner' or to give up on relationships when our dreams repeatedly don't match reality. An alternative is to regard the path of intimate relationship as 'relationship yoga', an ongoing spiritual practice and a process of unfolding and transformation.

In this chapter I introduce you to some profound Tantric meditations for couples that have the potential to offer you and your beloved a direct experience of being soulmates, of being ecstatic together, of finding Union. Before I describe these meditations, however, may I briefly remind you that the meditations in themselves won't do it for you. It is how you are in yourself, and to a lesser extent how your partner is in themselves, the distance that you have each travelled across your inner terrains, your capacity to be open to the present moment and the unpredictable winds of grace that will determine where the meditation takes you.

> *After all these years of Tantra, I felt lower than I ever had done. Larry and I had had a fight, and it seemed that for the last year or so, our sexual needs and desires had been completely at odds. Larry was sick of seeing me as a goddess and wanted a good fuck. I knew that the only way that I could have sex was when my heart was open, and there was an atmosphere of mutual respect and honouring. Where had all the bliss gone?*
>
> *I called a close girlfriend, one who I had known since the beginning of my Tantra days, and sobbed. I told her about all what I was finding painful and intolerable, and I knew that she understood. I was able to 'find myself' again. I found the courage to share with Larry how I was feeling, how vulnerable, scared and raw I felt. I expressed myself in my vulnerability and he heard me. Everything changed. And do you know what – a month later I'm happier than I ever have been! I should have known by now that life comes in waves, and that when I let myself sink to rock bottom, I bounce up again with renewed zest. For me, Tantra these days is less something that I do, and more something that I live. I don't need Larry to tell me that I'm a goddess to feel like one. I can trust in the wisdom of the Universe, even when it doesn't make sense. I can love when I feel hurt, and when I'm in the moment, miracles happen. This, to me, is ecstasy.*
>
> SANDRA, 44, SOCIAL WORKER

The heart wave and wave of bliss

The wave of bliss is a traditional Tantric meditation that facilitates energetic connection within yourself, between you and your partner, and ultimately with the Universe. It is best practised in stages, and I lead you through these. The heart wave, part one, is the foundation of the wave of bliss, and is also complete as a meditation in and of itself.

You will notice that in each stage of the heart wave and wave of bliss, Shakti leads. This is because in the iconography of Tantra, Shakti, the female principle or deity, represents pure energy, whereas Shiva, the male principle or deity, represents pure consciousness or form. Hence, Shakti, the woman, follows her flow of energy. Shiva, the man, matches it and gives it form. In fact, both men and women have masculine and feminine qualities and, in order to enhance their inner harmony, need to develop both capacities, of awareness and structure and of energy and flow. Ultimately, in the heart wave and the wave of bliss, there is no leading and following, but a blending, a melting. But we need to start somewhere, and this starting point, for some people (men in particular), can be a little unpalatable.

'Why should I let her lead?' asks one man. 'She's always trying to control me anyway.' In fact, this meditation is far, far removed from the whole arena of the battle of the sexes, or the power struggles in relationships. Neither Shakti nor Shiva are better or superior, and yet this definition of their specific roles can evoke impressions and images of such conflicts, when competition of this nature is alive, either openly or covertly, within the relationship. If this is the case for you, here lies an opportunity to reframe your perceptions and intentions to a cooperative approach. If you are not able or willing to cooperate at this moment, you get a chance to engage more deeply and to become more conscious of the nature and effects of your need to compete.

'But she breathes so slowly,' says another man, 'and I'd faint if I tried to match her breathing.' In fact, it is more common than not for two members of a couple to have different rhythms, in breathing and in life. Whereas this is an opportunity for Shiva to enter into Shakti's world, to explore her rhythm, Shakti too must be willing to be responsive to Shiva, and modify her rhythm if he's really struggling. Shakti, don't use your role to get even with Shiva. It's not a game to try to catch him out; it's an opportunity to meet more deeply. With the opening for intimacy also, as we have seen in Chapter 2, comes the potential for resistance. Both Shakti and Shiva need to take responsibility for their own attitudes, and to communicate honestly with each other if they are not in integrity.

I recommend that before practising these meditations, you take some time to arrive in a free and natural way in your body. You may begin with some kundalini shaking (*see page 53*), or else some free dancing. Loosen up your body and mind and find an easy sense of 'streaming', of energy flow through your body.

Enter in to these meditations with a lightness and playfulness. It is common for people who have a tendency to try hard and to want to get it right to become overly concerned with the mechanics of the exercise. In fact, however, the techniques themselves are simply the proverbial finger pointing to the moon. They are a means to an end, rather than an end in themselves, and struggling for perfection is actually less likely to get you there than a simple, relaxed presence.

The heart wave, part 1: meeting

The first part of the heart wave is about connecting within yourself, your love and sexuality, and then meeting with a partner from that place of harmony within yourself.

> #### The Technique
>
> Some gentle, rhythmic music such as *Tantric Sexuality* (*see* Resources, *page 250*) may be helpful. The meditation can take anything from ten minutes to half an hour, and you can practise it naked or clothed.
>
> - Sit opposite each other. Kneeling astride some cushions is ideal, as in this position your back is straight and your pelvis is free to move. Begin with a namaste

- Put the music on repeat, and close your eyes. Begin to breathe naturally, fully, in a relaxed and rhythmic way through your mouth. As you breathe out, rotate your pelvis forwards, as if gently thrusting with an energetic vajra. As you breathe in, rotate your pelvis back as if you are sucking energy into a vast and delicious yoni between your legs.

- Let your breath carry you. Find the ease and naturalness of this motion.

- As you inhale, squeeze your love muscle to whatever degree is comfortable for you.

- As you exhale, relax your love muscle.

- Again, find a relaxed and easy rhythm. Let the breathing, rocking and love muscle pulsations generate a charge in your pelvis. Place your awareness here. Become aware of your sexuality and the pleasure and energy that you are generating.

- When you feel in connection with your pelvis, open your eyes. Let your gaze be soft and receptive. When your partner opens their eyes, you can receive each other in this way, receiving also their sexual pleasure, and allowing yourself to be seen in yours.

- Take some time to really arrive together.

- When you feel that you have arrived, Shakti, begin to stroke your hand gently on your body, up and down with your breath. As you breathe in, stroke upwards from yoni to your heart. Imagine that you are breathing the pleasure in your pelvis into your heart, transforming it into love. As you breathe out, stroke downwards from your heart to your sex, bringing this love down into yoni.

- Shiva, begin to mirror Shakti, breathing in when she breathes in, breathing out when she breathes out, stroking from vajra to your heart as you inhale, and from heart to vajra as you exhale.

- Sense now this quality of meeting: meeting in the heart and meeting in the sex. You can imagine that as you breathe and stroke up to your heart you are silently saying 'here I am in my love' and as you breathe and stroke down to your sex, imagine silently saying a phrase to the effect of 'Here I am in my sexuality.'

- Remember to stay in touch with yourself. If you find that you are thinking or losing touch with yourself, close your eyes for a while until you reconnect.

- Don't look for fireworks. Just relax into the simplicity of this experience of connection with yourself and meeting with your partner.

- If you are not feeling particularly loving or are not experiencing much pleasure in your pelvis, don't worry. Welcome how you feel and enter more deeply into it. It is normal, for example, as the heart opens more, to experience some tears of grief. Notice whatever is present in you, rather than looking for what is not. Relax into what is here. Do not try to analyse or understand. Underneath all feelings felt deeply and let go of is love. When we are fully present in our love and in our sexuality, and allow ourselves to meet from that place, this is a deeply intimate experience.

- When you feel that it is the right time to complete, let go of the stroking and again just breathe and rock together, with or without the love muscle, in eye contact. Then close your eyes and give yourself your full attention. Feel and notice what is happening inside you.

> - Open your eyes when you are ready. Share a namaste and take some time to embrace or cuddle and to share your experiences.

How were your experiences of the heart wave, part one? Remember that there is no right or wrong way to experience this, or any other meditation. The meditation is here to show you more about yourself, and what happens energetically inside you as you enter into the exercise. Below are some common difficulties encountered in this meditation, and an explanation of what their origins may be.

Some people find that they do not experience pleasure in their pelvis when they begin the meditation. Hopefully, by now you will be familiar with your love muscle, and will have some experiences and ideas of how your pelvic floor is structured energetically. If you are holding pain in your love muscle, it will reappear whatever you do, until you have healed it. Remember to be patient with yourself, as healing can be a gradual and ongoing process.

Alternatively, you may feel frustration and not much pleasure if you have become caught up in 'doing it right'. If this is the case, you may like to take a break from the meditation and consider how trying to 'do it right' has affected your life and your sexual relationships. Then loosen up – do some kundalini shaking or dancing, express with your voice your frustration or sadness. Let your energy move. When you feel clearer, resume the meditation. If you repeatedly get stuck in this attitude of performance, you might try to let go of some of the components of the meditation. For example, forget about the love muscle. Even forget about the rocking if you're still stuck. Focus on really receiving your partner and your experiences in each moment, as you gaze into each other's eyes. When this is natural for you, gradually introduce the other components.

One of the greatest opponents of pleasure, love and ecstasy is expectation. Do not expect to reach nirvana. Focus more on reaching a place in yourself where you experience you, as you are, with as much openness in your body, heart and mind as is available for you. Then practise doing the same with receiving your partner. As I have written earlier, self-awareness breeds self-acceptance, which can blossom into self-love. These qualities are the foundation of all Tantric practice, both in terms of your capacity to truly love your beloved for who they really are, and in terms of opening to ecstasy and transcendent states of awareness.

> *This intensifies the feeling of closeness to Mike; it raises deep emotions every time. I usually want to cry ... with happiness.*
>
> CARALYN, 38, MOTHER

The heart wave, part 2: exchange

The second part of the heart wave extends the energetic meeting into an energetic exchange.

The Technique

- Begin as for the heart wave, part one, and continue through all the stages up to the meeting at heart and sex.

- When you have a sense of meeting each other in a clear and loving way, Shiva, on an in-breath, hold your breath, your hand and your awareness in your heart. Shakti, you do not hold your breath. As you exhale, continue to stroke down your body from heart to sex. When you reach your sex, however, do not stop there. Continue exhaling, and with your hand extend the energy of your sexuality out of your sex and into that of Shiva's, as shown in the illustration (*see below*). Continue with your hand up, just in front of Shiva's body, to his heart, meeting his hand there.

- Now Shiva, as Shakti inhales, you exhale, and move your hand with hers, almost touching, about an inch away. Feel and sense the space between your hand and hers, imagining an invisible connection between them. As you breathe out and down to your sex, also continue your exhalation as you extend your hand and your energy from your sex into Shakti's and up to her heart. Continue in this way, breathing and moving in a U-shaped arc, breathing alternately, one breath for each journey from heart to heart.

- Although your hands move outside of your own and your partner's body, imagine that your energy is entering into them, and that their energy is entering into you. This is an energy exchange.

- Become particularly attentive to the moment of entering, energetically, into your partner's body, and to the moment of them entering you. In this meditation, you alternately experience both your penetrative potential, as you energetically enter the genitals of your partner, and your receptive potential, as you receive them. Distinctions of male and female can fall away.

- When you are ready to complete, let go of the hand movements and simply breathe and move together (however it comes) in eye contact.

- Then close your eyes and sense what is still moving, what you feel and sense inside yourself, as gradually and naturally your body comes to rest.

- End with a namaste, and take some time to embrace or cuddle and share your experiences.

> Breath exchange brings me a beautiful sense of merging with Caralyn. It is possibly as intimate as genital penetration.
>
> MIKE, 42, COMPUTER ANALYST

The wave of bliss, part 1: meditation

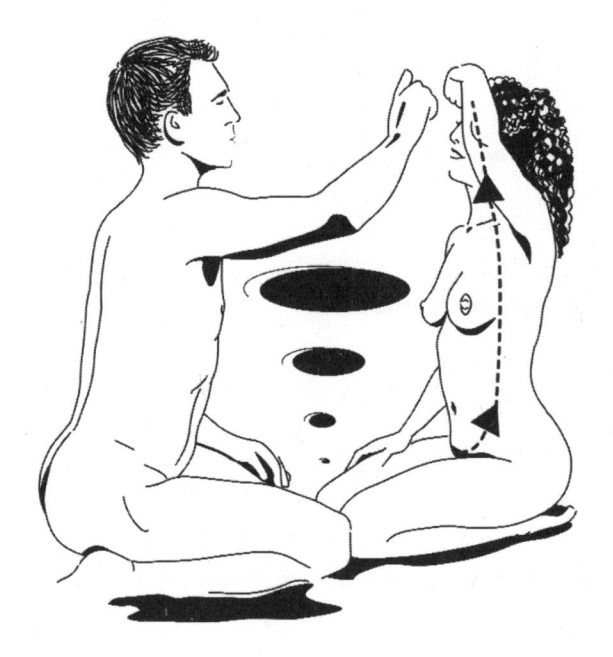

STROKE UP YOUR BODY TO YOUR THIRD EYE

The wave of bliss is an extension of part one of the heart wave that includes the third eye, centre of consciousness and bliss. This meditation is not an energy-building cycle, as is the male-female breath (*see page 143*), but a gently deepening one. There is a constant dynamo of charge in the genitals, from where the energy is distributed, transformed and harmonised within each person, and exchanged between the two. The swinging of the energy, the breathing and the connection with the third eye leads to a profound relaxation, and a merging of the boundaries between Shakti and Shiva.

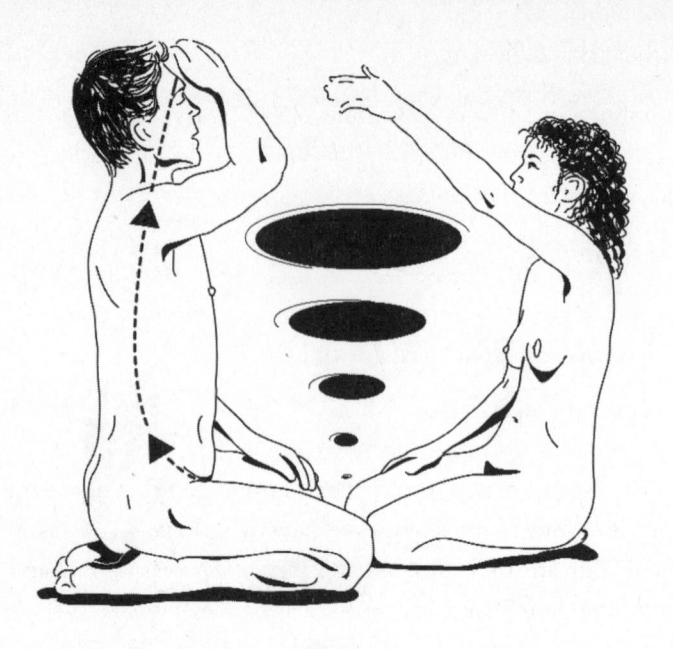

MIRROR THE MOVEMENT FOR SHAKTI

The Technique

Allow around twenty to thirty minutes for this part of the meditation.

- Begin with a namaste, and continue with the heart wave, part one (*see page 235*), until you sense a clear meeting. Do not proceed to the heart wave, part two.

- While still breathing together, or synchronously, Shakti, on an in-breath, stroke up your body, to your heart, and beyond up to your third eye. As you exhale, breathe and stroke down to your sex. Continue breathing between your sex and third eye, being aware of each movement flowing through and including your heart.

- Shiva, mirror Shakti, breathing between sex and third eye, through your heart.

- Continue in this way for a while. Shakti, you can experiment with holding your breath and holding your hand, thus holding the energy up at your third eye. When you do this, Shiva does the same. This intensifies the experience of your own third eye, and of meeting in this place. You can intersperse holding the energy at your third eye with breathing normally, up and down, between your third eye and sex.

- Whenever you are ready, Shiva, you initiate the change from synchronous breathing (an energetic meeting) to alternate breathing (an energetic exchange). In a similar manner to the way it is done in the heart wave, part two (*see page 239*), you hold your breath, your hand and your awareness up in your third eye. You Shakti, carry on exhaling. Your out-breath no longer ends at your sex, but extends out from here and into Shiva's sex, up, just above his body, through his heart area to his third eye, to meet his hand there.

- At this point, you, Shiva, exhale, and yours and Shakti's hands move together as one, without physically touching, down through your body, out and into Shakti's, and up to her third eye. Continue with this U-shaped movement of energy, and let yourself sink more and more deeply into it.

- Before you complete this meditation, let go of the hand movements, and breathe and rock together in eye contact. Sense and feel the energy still swinging between you.

- When you are ready, close your eyes and feel the energy moving within you. Notice whatever you sense or feel inside your body. Gradually come to rest and open your eyes.

- Receive your beloved once more with your gaze, and complete with a namaste.

- Take a few moments to share your experiences.

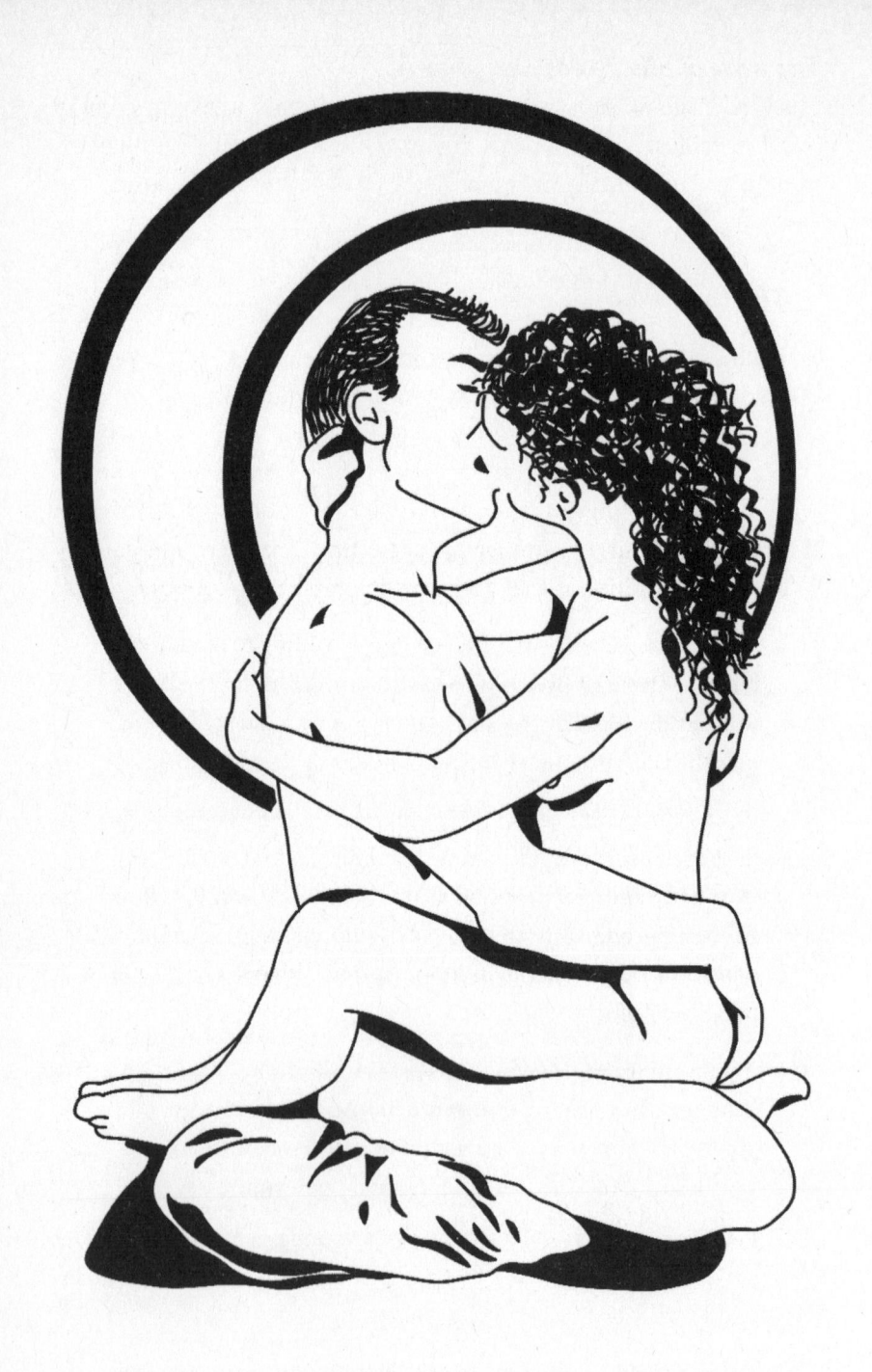

THE WAVE OF BLISS

The wave of bliss, part 2: expansion

The final stage of the wave of bliss is best practised in the position of 'yab-yum', illustrated opposite. You may do this with or without penetration, as a meditation in and of itself, or as part of lovemaking.

The Technique

In this state of meditation, time is irrelevant. You may spend anything from ten minutes to an hour in meditation.

In yab-yum, Shiva sits cross-legged and Shatkti sits in his lap. Your genitals will touch, and vajra can enter yoni. If you are not comfortable in this position, you can try variations such as Shiva sitting in a chair, or with legs outstretched. The main component of this position is that both partners' spines are upright.

- Begin as in the wave of bliss, part one (*see page 242*), up to the point of alternate breathing between sex, heart and third eye, without the hand movements. Alternatively, make love, come into the yab-yum position, and continue as described below.

- In yab-yum, continue breathing alternately and moving in this U-shaped exchange, indicating the energetic movements with your body and breath, rather than with your hands. It may at first appear odd, as both your pelvises move together in the same direction, rather than in the 'normal' lovemaking movement of in and out.

- After a while, let your foreheads touch each other, as you close your eyes. Just feel the energy swinging between you.

- When you have found a deep place of meditation, move on to exchanging your breath. Open your mouths, and place your lips together, forming an airtight seal. Feel the exchange of your breath. As your beloved exhales, you inhale their breath. As you exhale, your breath enters your beloved.

- At this point, your visualisation changes. Shakti, as you breathe in, breathe in and up from your sex, to your heart and up to your mouth. As you breathe out, imagine your energy entering into your beloved and descending through their body to their sex. Shiva, as you breathe in, now breathe in Shakti's breath through her mouth, and take it into you and down, through your heart, to your sex. Breathe out from your sex into hers, and up through her body to her mouth. You are now moving your energy in a circle. Relax deeply into it. Sense, feel or imagine this circle of oneness.

- Let yourself melt. You may feel, Shakti, that Shiva's vajra is reaching right up through you to your heart and beyond, filling you with a scintillating flow.

- Shiva, you may have a sense of penetrating Shakti deeply, and her love and the 'golden rain' of life energy raining down upon you.

- You may loose the sense of your separateness, of your gender, of your form. You may be filled with bliss, peace, silence. You may have a sense of the Universe.

- When your meditation comes to a natural place of completion, rest for a while together in silence, share a namaste and then share your experiences in words.

> *We had spent time giving and receiving pleasure, and I felt a wonderful moist aliveness in my yoni. The giving and receiving of pleasure without orgasm had awakened a tender intimacy between us. I knew that James completely respected my boundaries, and would ask, either verbally or with his eyes, before making the slightest move. He was very soft inside himself, open, and at times his eyes were moist. This*

gave me the safety to be soft myself. I can't have an experience like this with a macho man; even though we can have great sex and I can have good orgasms, the experience is totally different.

Our breathing rhythm was matched, and we were moving. He had his hand on yoni and we were gently tracing the flow of our breath with our fingers, stroking up his body, down his body, up mine, and down again. I felt his subtle body coming into mine, like a symbolic penis, through this breathing, and enhanced by the touch. And it was balanced. At other moments, I had an energetic penis and he had an energetic vagina, so our energies were equal. This added to my feelings of openness because he let me into him on an energetic level. This lasted a long time – I don't know exactly how long, but at least half an hour, which was wonderful. At the beginning I thought of it just as an exercise, but after a while I relaxed more and started really being and experiencing.

I hadn't had sex for a long time, because of a very early menopause, and I had lost my libido and didn't even know if I could become aroused, or how. This experience brought all of my energies and juices back. I could feel my womb opening up, and this opening reached all the way up to my heart, which felt as if it was swelling. This happened quite gradually, through the rhythmic deep breathing and the finger stroking. It felt as if we were on the same frequency. It was as if this symbolic penis was growing inwards and upwards. When it reached my third chakra, I became even softer. I can have good 'hard sex' where my third chakra doesn't have to open, but here the softness touched me. This allowed my heart to really open. I felt a lot of love for James, but in me. It was my love. The eye contact was also very important. I could really see him; not just his face, but his heart and soul too. I suppose this was my third eye opening.

I felt orgasmic the whole time. It wasn't like 'having an

orgasm', and yet I was so close to it for so long. And then it didn't stop. It just stayed, vibrating gently inside me. I had read about experiences such as these, but it was the first time that I had felt it. I felt as if I had had an orgasm, and yet it was still happening. When I got up I had wobbly legs, and it was difficult to think straight, just like after an orgasm.

I knew that if the energy had come all the way up and out of the top of my head, I would have had a 'Universal Orgasm'. But I didn't go there. I wasn't ready. It still took me a while to digest this, what I would call a 'spiritual orgasm', and I was still gently buzzing for days afterwards.

DOMINIQUE, 42, TRANSLATOR

Do not look for a transcendent experience, as this will, almost certainly, prevent one from occurring. Whatever your experience is, let it be, and embrace it. It may be a 'peak experience', a gentle sense of well-being or a deeper experience of your resistances to letting go and opening up. Either way, this is where you are meant to be! Remember too that you can return to exercises and meditations outlined earlier in the book, to support you in facing and letting go of resistances. Remember too that most people need the support of an understanding Tantric friend, or an experienced Tantric practitioner, at some point in their Tantric journey. Tantra is non-linear. It is not about getting somewhere, but about celebrating the path, which eventually leads you back to the place where you first started, but a different you. So you might as well enjoy the ride!

AFTER ENLIGHTENMENT, CHOPPING WOOD

As the Zen saying goes, before enlightenment, chopping wood; after enlightenment, chopping wood. Life goes on as before, and yet everything has changed. I am not suggesting that by now you are enlightened – far from it – but you may have tasted ecstasy. As I am sure is abundantly clear to you now, Tantra is far more than a collection of techniques for improving your sex life. Don't let your experience of ecstasy, bliss or enjoyment of life be confined to the bedroom: bring it into the whole of your life! As you come full circle and go to work, look after the children and cook, bring an awareness of sexy deliciousness into whatever you do.

> *It may sound rather dramatic and over the top, but, nonetheless, it is true to say that Tantra has changed my life for the better in no uncertain terms. There is not one single relationship in my life that hasn't benefited, be it as a lover, a friend, a sister, a daughter, a work colleague and, perhaps most importantly, my relationship with me.*
>
> ANNIE, 38, VIDEO PRODUCER

In the Native American creation myth, Grandfather Sun made love with Grandmother Earth, and created Earth Beings. If we look carefully, we can see evidence of the sexual-spiritual union of male and female principles everywhere. Even computers are plugged together by means of male and female sockets. Nature blooms with sexuality; birdsong is a mating call. Let life awaken the joy of creation within you, and remember to celebrate yourself!

RESOURCES

Books: Tantra

Anand, Margot, *The Art of Everyday Ecstasy: The Seven Tantric Keys for Bringing Passion, Spirit and Joy into Every Part of Your Life*, Piatkus Books, 1998.
Odier, Daniel, *Tantric Quest*, Inner Traditions International, 1997.
Odier, Daniel, *Desire: The Tantric Path to Awakening*, Inner Traditions International, 2001.
Osho, *Meditation: The First and Last Freedom*, available from Osho Purnima Distribution, Greenwise, Vange Pk Rd, Basildon, Essex, SS16 5LA. Tel: 01268 584 141.
Richardson, Diana, *The Love Keys*, HarperCollins, 1999.
Sampson, Val, *Tantra: The Art of Mindblowing Sex*, Vermilion, 2002.
Shaw, Miranda, *Passionate Enlightenment: Women in Tantric Buddhism*, Princeton University Press, 1995.

Books: Related Subjects

Duffell, Nick and Lovendal, Helena, *Love, Sex and the Dangers of Intimacy*, HarperCollins, 2002.
Gibran, Kahlil, *The Prophet*, Wordsworth Classics of World Literature, 1996.
Heskell, Peta, *The Flirt Coach's Guide to Finding the Love You Want: Communication Tips for Relationship Success*, HarperCollins, 2003.
Myss, Caroline, *Anatomy of the Spirit: The Seven Stages of Power and Healing*, Bantam, 1997.
Oriah Mountain Dreamer, *The Invitation*, HarperCollins, 2000.
Ram Dass, *One Liners: A Mini-Manual for a Spiritual Life*, Piatkus, 2003.
Richardson, Cheryl, *Take Time for Your Life*, Bantam, 2002.
Rosenberg, Marshall, *Non-violent Communication*, Independent Publishers' Group, 2003.
Some, Sobonfu, *The Spirit of Intimacy: Ancient Teachings in the Ways of Relationships*, Quill, 2000.

Spoken word audio cassettes: Tantra

Lightwoman, Leora, *Diamond Light Tantra: Opening to Pleasure, Love and Ecstasy*, Recorded lecture at Alternatives, 2001. Available from Diamond Light Tantra shop, www.diamondlighttantra.com, Tel: 08700 780 584.
Long, Barry, *Making Love: Sexual Love the Divine Way*, Barry Long Books, 1996.

Spoken word audio cassettes: Related Subjects

Spezzano, Chuck, *The Psychology of Vision* series, available from www.psychologyofvision.com
Ram Dass tapes. Available from Living Dharma Tapes, Poulstone Court, Kings Caple, Herefordshire HR1 4UA. livingdharma@btinternet.com

Music

Mellow /Tantric:
Llewellyn with Leora Lightwoman, *Tantric Sexuality* (includes introductory booklet), New World Music, www.newworldmusic.com, also available from Diamond Light Tantra shop, www.diamondlighttantra.com.
Klaus Weise, *el-HADRA: The Mystic Dance*.
Vangelis, *Voices*.

Earthy:
Charlie McMahon, *Tjilatjila* (gentle).
James Asher, *Feet in the Soil* (energetic).
Frank Natale, *Shaman's Breath* (very energetic). Available from www.franknatale.com

Other:
Baka Beyond, *The Meeting Pool* (playful, childlike).
Sash, *Encore Une Fois* (dance music).

Specific Meditations:
Awakening the Energy Body. Includes guided Kundalini Shaking plus two other Tantric meditations. Available from Diamond Light Tantra shop, www.diamondlighttantra.com, tel: 08700 780 584.
Chakra Breathing Meditation. Available from Osho Purnima Distribution (see books section for details).
Kundalini Meditation, Osho Purnima Distribution (as above).
Michael Shrieve, *Transfer Station Blue* (for Kundalini Shaking).

Video

Leora Lightwoman and Roger Lichy, *Tantric Sexuality*. Available from New World Music (see music section for details) and Diamond Light Tantra shop.

Diamond Light Tantra shop

Stocks a range of Leora Lightwoman's spoken word/meditation/music audio cassettes and CDs, videos, her books, and related products. Details and ordering from www.diamondlighttantra.com. Tel: 08700 780 584.

Tantra Workshops

Diamond Light Tantra workshops with Leora Lightwoman
Tel: 08700 780 584
www.diamondlighttantra.com
info@diamondlighttantra.com

Products

Eros lubricants. Available from www.eros-uk.co.uk or tel: 01672 520 123. (Ideally use a silicone-based variety for vajra pleasuring, as it doesn't dry up, and a water-based one for yoni and lovemaking.)

INDEX

'admiring yoni' exercise 188–90
affairs 76
altars 41, 45, 46
appreciations 68–9
attention 80–1
awareness 79–82
'awareness in life' exercise 80

'back-to-back dance' 32–5
baths 152
beauty, creating 20
belief systems, limiting 171–3
blended pleasuring 221
bliss 173–6
body
    awareness of 79–82
    fully inhabiting xiv
    love of 150–8
boundaries 6–7, 102, 106–8, 159, 161–7, 184
breasts 133, 183–7, 220
    breast cancer 184
    breast massage 184–6
    breast meditation 186–7
breathing 8, 85–90
    see also heart wave exercise; wave of bliss exercise
    chakra breathing 117–25, 215
    full body exercise 86–9

cancer, breast 184
Chakra Breathing (CD) 118–22, 124
chakras (energy centres) 8, 79, 100–14
    base/first 103–4, 116, 120, 121, 206
    chakra breathing meditation 117–25, 215
    chakra talk 125–7
    crown/seventh 103, 112–14, 122, 206
    definition 100–1
    health 101–3
    heart/fourth 103, 108–9, 127, 135
    meeting 115–27

    sacral/second 103, 105–6, 121–2
    solar plexus/third 103, 106–8, 122, 182
    third eye/sixth 26, 64, 103, 111–12, 241–3
    throat/fifth 103, 109–11
change, fear of 15–18
childhood experience 71–2, 90, 112–13, 131–2, 158
childhood masturbation 208–9
childhood sexual abuse 44, 102, 107, 134
clitoris 189, 221
communication 66–9, 109–11
competition, between women 178–82
connectedness 2, 3, 63, 123, 144, 160
control, letting go of 232
coughs 110–11

dances
    see also kundalini shaking
    'back-to-back dance' 32–5
    'dance of freedom and togetherness' 73–7
    'distancer-pursuer' dance 69–73
    'fingertip heart dance' 35–9
Deep Diving Tantra 70, 193, 215, 231
deep listening 66–8
defining Tantra xi–xv
dependence 194
Diamond Light Tantra 57, 58
diary keeping 11, 152–3
discomfort, with Tantric exercises 32–3
'distancer-pursuer dance' 69–73

ecstasy 52, 230–2, 238–9, 248–9
ejaculation
    female 224
    postponing male 173, 224, 225, 227
emotional expression 96
empowerment, between women 178–82
energetic blocks 78–9, 140
energy body 100, 176
    see also chakras (energy centres)

252 — Index

energy flow, gender differences 128–48
erogenous zones 184
exercises xix–xx
    see also specific exercises
expansion 79, 99, 176
expectations, disengaging from 19–20
'expressive sound' meditation 95–6
'eye (soul) gazing' 64–6

father-son relationship 195–7
'female breath' exercise 137–40
female energy flow 129, 133–4, 137–48
female sexuality 177–92
'female-male breath' exercise 141–6
feminine energy
    of men 234
    of women 85, 146–8
'fingertip heart dance' 35–9
food 41, 44–5
free dancing 91, 234, 238
freedom 75, 148

genitals 208–28
    see also vajra (penis); yoni (vagina)
God 112–14
God/Goddess within 33, 45, 233
    see also Shakti; Shiva
goddess spot 221, 222
grounding 58–9, 119

healing, sexual xv–xvi, 193–5
heart 36–8
'heart wave' exercise 234–41
Heaven and Earth meditation 104
hedonism 160
homophobia 193–4
homosexuality 146–7, 199

identity 195
impotence 132
initiation rites, sexual 177
inner child, playful 92
inner flute 102
'inner lover' meditation 48–51
intention 20–1, 82–5
intimacy 30, 60–77, 163

kundalini meditation 56
kundalini shaking 53–8, 91, 135, 137, 234, 238

lesbians 146–7
'liberating sexual energy' exercise 51–8
listening skills 66–8
love
    opening to 149–59
    and sex 35–6, 39, 128–32, 134, 141, 163
love (pelvic floor) muscles 116–17, 222, 236, 237, 238
lubricants 218, 220–1, 225

macho-ness 132

'male breath' exercise 132, 133, 135–7
male energy flow 128–33, 135–7, 140–8, 204–7
male sexuality 193–207
'male-female breath' exercise 141–6
marriage, as inner death 83
marriage proposals 71
masculine energy, of women 85, 146–8, 234
massage 198–202
    all-over-body 219
    breast 184–6
    genital 216–18
masturbation 208–14
meditation 11, 91–6
    see also heart wave exercise; wave of bliss exercise
    breast meditation 186–7
    chakra breathing meditation 117–25, 215
    Heaven and Earth meditation 104
    inner lover meditation 48–51
    kundalini meditation 56
    receptive gaze 63
    Tantric touch exercise 173–6
    vajra meditations 202–6
    yin-yang 167–71
    yoni gazing 190–2
'melting hug' exercise 28–31
mentors 21
mirrors, other people as 22–3, 60–2, 123, 179
moment-by-moment awareness iv, 81, 215
mother-infant relationship 23, 194–5
movement 90–4

nakedness 7, 151–2, 154–7
namaste (heart salutation) 11, 15, 22–7, 62, 229
Native American tradition 249
nature 63
needs 68
New Men 129
no, learning to say 74, 75, 161–7

oneness/wholeness 40, 48, 60, 160, 230
oral sex 218
orgasms 104, 173, 231–2, 246, 247–8
    absence 2, 85
    multiple-orgasms 218–28
    through chakra breathing 124–5
    through masturbation 214
    valley orgasm 227
    whole-body orgasm 8
origins of Tantra xii
Osho's Anger Meditation 91

parents, unloving 52
pelvic floor (love) muscles 116–17, 222, 236, 237, 238
'pelvic rocking' meditation 92–4
pelvis 32, 33–5, 38, 120, 236
penis see vajra
perineum 227

pleasure 215–18
  opening to 160–76
pleasure bridge 225
pleasuring, blended 221
prayer position 26
pregnancy 184
punctuality 22–3

receptive gaze 62–4
relationships
  caring for 12, 13
  intimate as spiritual path 60–77
  phases 5
  relationship yoga 232–48
relaxation 97–8
reparenting yourself 196–7
resistance 15–18

sacred space 10, 15, 18–21
sacredness 230
scent 41, 43
self
  caring for 13
  getting to know 74–5
  mirrored in other people 22–3, 60–2, 123, 179
self-acceptance/awareness 149–50
self-love 149–59
sensitivity, awakening 176
sensuality
  as gateway to the Spirit 40, 161
  reconnecting with 7–8
  sensory awakening ritual 40–6
  whole-body 32
separation-individuation 194–5
sex, and love 35–6, 39, 128–32, 134, 141, 163
sex drive
  incompatible drives 70
  unleashing 4–5
sexual abuse 44, 102, 107, 134
sexual development xv–xvi
sexual energy, liberating 51–8
sexual frustration 76–7
sexual healing xv–xvi, 193–5
'Shah!' exercise 107–8, 178–82
Shakti xii, xvii, 73, 152, 190–1, 216, 218–24, 226–8, 234–7, 239–46
shame 158–9, 209
Shiva xii, xvi, 73, 152, 190–1, 193, 204, 216, 218–24, 234–5, 239–46
showers 152
sight 41, 45–6
silence 124
single people 4, 5, 47–59
  namaste 23–4, 25
  workshops 5, 6–7
sound 41, 42–3, 95–7, 121
  see also 'Shah!' exercise
  releasing in Kundalini shaking 55
  in sex 96–7

Spirit 40, 158, 161

taboos 210
Tantras xii
Tantric dates 10, 11–18, 27
Tantric principles 78–99
'Tantric touch' exercise 173–6
Tantrikas (Tantric practitioners) 6, 9, 11
taste 41, 43–4
Temple of the Spirit xiv
tension 97
terminology xvi–xvii
third being 165
third eye 26, 64, 103, 111–12, 241, 242–3
time management 13
tiredness, as resistance 16
touch 8
  see also massage
  nervousness about 31
  non-sexual between men 197–202
  working on your sense of 41, 44–5

union 73, 229–49
unity xiii
Universe/Universal 229, 230, 233, 246

vagina see yoni
vajra (penis) xvi, 89, 199, 224–8, 229, 236
  awareness of 81
  energy flow 129–30, 135–7, 141, 143–4
  love muscle exercises 116
  massage 216–17
  masturbation 210, 212–13
  relaxing 98
  vajra gazing 215
  vajra meditation 202–4
  vajra root meditation 205–6
vibrators 210

wants 167–71
wave of bliss exercises 234–5, 241–8
womb 105–6
workshops 5–9, 57
  see also Deep Diving Tantra; Diamond Light Tantra

yab-yum posture 123, 124, 244–5
'yes, no, maybe and please' exercise 163–7
yin-yang meditation 167–71
yoga 1
  relationship yoga 232–48
yoni (vagina) xvi, 85, 220–3, 229, 236
  admiring 188–90
  awareness of 81
  energy flow 133–4, 138–9, 140–1, 143–4
  love muscle exercises 116
  massage 216–17
  masturbation 210, 212–13
  relaxing 98
  yoni gazing 190–2, 215
  yoni wisdom 187–92